My Secret Life with a Sex Addict

From Discovery to Recovery
by

Emma Dawson, M.S.W., L.C.S.W.

*Thanks to my daughters and friends,
personal and professional,
who supported and encouraged me
to tell my story.*

Foreword

Life brings us countless joys. What many of our parents didn't tell us is that life also brings many painful tests and wrenching heartbreaks. One of life's most difficult challenges is to encounter sexual addiction in an intimate relationship. Without any familiarity with this disorder, addiction can firmly grip a person, just as it grips the partner. The co-addict becomes addicted to the addict, his behavior and his emotional turmoil, and tries to change and control both him and the confounding beast that rules his life.

The dance begins. "I'll lend all my energy to fix him. I'll improve myself to be more appealing. I'll do whatever it takes to make him happy. Never mind the emotional cost — anything to hold onto him, to avoid looking the beast in the eye, to confront what it might say about me, about him, about our family."

Sexual addiction has been the subject of debate for many years. The fields of psychology and psychiatry did not formally recognize its existence for years. Since sexual addiction was not recognized, sex addicts were not inclined to step forward. Their experience was denied. Thus, the addict was relegated to the shadows feeling alienated, misunderstood, hopeless and ashamed.

And what about the co-dependent spouse? Her secret is even more removed from common awareness. She is left to stand alone, feeling bewildered and inadequate, while languishing in embarrassment and resentment. Clinicians have often said that, while the pain of the addict is immense, few can fully appreciate the frequently greater anguish of the co-addict.

Emma Dawson has stepped forward to break the secrecy that surrounds sexual addiction and co-addiction. Courageously, she reveals her personal struggle to understand how her husband's addiction was not about her and not about any personal inadequacy. Dawson validates the experience of millions of Americans who have lived with sexual addiction. *My Secret Life with a Sex Addict* lifts the partner guilt that accompanies this insidious disorder and all its accompanying denial. This important book offers both understanding and hope. It will begin the healing process for many. Sensitively written, Dawson's first book not only teaches us much about sexual addiction, it also confirms there is a way out.

Many have suffered, but many have also grown. With every one of life's tests, there is a hidden gift. The task is to discover those treasures that reside within and let the legacy of sexual addiction be one of growth and transformation.

Geral Blanchard, MA, LPC
co-author *Sexual Abuse in America: Epidemic of the 21st Century*

About the Author

The author of *MY SECRET LIFE WITH A SEX ADDICT: FROM DISCOVERY TO RECOVERY,* Emma Dawson is a recovered victim of her ex-husband's sexual addiction. She was in a 29-year marriage with an addict whose behavior became progressively worse. Since terminating her marriage, she completed a Master's Degree in Social Work, become a Licensed Clinical Social Worker and gained experience in the field. Emma has worked as a social worker in a psychiatric hospital and has experience in family, group and individual outpatient therapy.

Discovering little has been published about sexual addiction, written from the spouse's point of view, prompted Emma Dawson to write this book.

Table of Contents

	12	Introduction
	15	Prologue
Chapter I	17	Secrets Revealed
Chapter II	27	Testing the Secrets
Chapter III	45	The Secrets Begin
Chapter IV	59	Secrets I Kept from Myself
Chapter V	77	Family Secrets
Chapter VI	93	Sharing the Secrets with Others
Chapter VII	109	Discovering the Secrets of Dreams
Chapter VIII	119	My Secrets to Beginning the Healing Journey as a Single Person
Chapter IX	126	Lessons Learned from My Secrets
	137	Epilogue
	139	Symptoms

Introduction

As I sought to educate myself about sex addiction, I learned that its potential for devastation is at least as strong as that of other, more familiar addictions, such as drug, gambling or alcohol addiction. A diagnosis of sex addiction is dependent on whether the behavior is destructive, persistent and escalating. The addiction can manifest itself in masturbation, pornography, prostitution, exhibitionism, voyeurism, indecent phone calls, multiple sexual partners, child molestation, rape and even violence. There are estimated to be 16,000,000 people who exhibit these behaviors to relieve their inner pain and anxiety. These addicts are attempting to manage feelings of anger, loneliness and emptiness. Those who are in a relationship with such addicts will find them to be selfish, needy and preoccupied. This book offers samples of these behaviors.

The most informative book I found on the subject of sex addiction was Patrick Carnes' *Out of the Shadows: Understanding Sexual Addiction*, 1983 edition. Carnes defines an addiction or dependency as the mood altering attachment to sexual thoughts, rituals and behaviors resulting in severe stress to the addict and the family. The need for a sexual fix becomes more important than family, friends, work and values — as deadly as any chemical addiction and more difficult to recognize. Violent mood swings may be a reaction of the addict to the shame of compulsive activity he really doesn't want. Having sex with those he doesn't know or even like is another indicator. Finally, if a person is unable to stop engaging in behavior which absolutely contradicts his or her own deepest values, he or she almost certainly suffers from a sex addiction.

I heard Ted say and do things that confirmed his sex addiction. He progressed through several levels of risky behavior. I was incredulous as he began to reveal years of secret activities as a sex addict. When he told me of his many heterosexual encounters, he concluded with, "If I could go three weeks without having a sexual encounter with someone I would tell myself that I did not have a problem." He continued, "I didn't even like some of the women." He was a man who did not want to continue his behavior but could not control it.

I had no idea he was making obscene phone calls to women within the first seven years of our marriage. One behavior I did observe was his interest in watching the lighted bathroom and bedroom windows of our neighbor's house from the pool in our backyard. His voyeurism could have led to an arrest and prosecution if the victim had observed him. The women who received his obscene phone calls were also victims.

He ultimately confessed to having many heterosexual relationships with employees, friends, strangers, colleagues and acquaintances. If he had been exposed and charged with sexual harassment by employees or colleagues in the company, it could have cost him his job and jeopardized his career. He was risking his health and mine by exposing himself to sexually transmitted diseases such as AIDS, from strangers and acquaintances. He had exploited many of these women to fulfill his need for a sexual fix. When he revealed this information to me I lost trust and respect, and was unable to regain it.

I, too, felt exploited when our lovemaking became mechanical. The nurturing, growing and life-enhancing aspects of a sexual relationship were sacrificed. It was demoralizing to feel like an object — finally realizing I was another victim of his addiction.

Most devastating for me was my discovery of the years of sexual abuse suffered by one of our beautiful and beloved daughters. She confided in me well after her departure from home and her parents' divorce. Her father's behavior created yet another high-risk situation for him because of the extreme potential for legal consequences. He could have been charged with incest in the early stages of her abuse had she gone to authorities or confided in me.

My husband's behaviors could have cost him his family, his job, his career and his health, but nothing deterred him. The addiction had control of his life.

Prologue

"Me? You've got to be insane!" With that my husband stalked from the room. Just diagnosed as a sex addict, he was angry with the therapist and highly offended by the label. When he came home and told me, I had a million questions. I had never heard the term "sexual addiction" and knew nothing about its implications.

I was not alone in being uneducated about this syndrome. Many people reacted to the term "sex addict" with ignorance, misunderstanding and even cruelty. Some laughed at me as though I was being facetious. It made me feel like a fool when I so wanted and needed some compassion. I still brace myself when I use the term. Perhaps the most common reaction is what I call the "titter response." Both men and women will snicker, "That sounds like fun!" or "You mean you're complaining?" Men will often comment "More power to him!" There also is an assumption that the partner of the sex addict must be sexually inadequate, or perhaps that the addict indulges in a variety of "kinky" behaviors. Because of our cultural admiration of sexual prowess, sex addiction is often viewed as a desirable affliction.

On the contrary, sex addiction is anything but desirable. It encompasses a syndrome of destructive behaviors that can demolish marriages, families and lives. In today's world it is also physically dangerous.

It is time to share the story I hope will be helpful to other spouses or significant others of sex addicts. This is my own story, detailing my experiences and expressing my feelings frankly and fully, so that people in similar situations may compare them with their own.

At the beginning of our turbulent times, I began recording my thoughts, feelings and recollections of our conversations. In this book, my focus is on my personal experience and my feelings as I struggled to define and understand them. The story is also intended to help others identify, understand and solve the dilemma of having a relationship with an addict, particularly a sex addict. The education and clinical experience I have acquired as a Licensed Clinical Social Worker enhance my story. Since facing my husband's sex addiction, I worked my way through feelings of despair and hopelessness to a point of tranquility, acceptance and optimism. I hope that my story will provide a confrontation with the reality of sexual addiction, as well as provide the comfort of knowing there are ways to be healed. I invite you along as I share my story of discovery and recovery from an abusive relationship.

All of the facts and events in this book are true. The names and identities of the spouses and other persons have been changed. The locales have been moved to New York.

Chapter I

Secrets Revealed

"What would happen if one woman told the truth about her life? The world would split open." — *Muriel Rukeyser*

I had done an excellent job of keeping the truth from myself, but it had to come out eventually. Ted and I were living with so much tension that an explosion was virtually inevitable. The blast would tear apart the barriers I had erected between myself and reality. Sadly, ironically, it was Mother's Day when the explosion came that first began to uncover for me Ted's secret life.

The week before Mother's Day, in the 28th year of marriage, bore signs of the impending explosion. Ted had been arriving home late more and more often. His pattern was to arrive, glance at the mail quickly, then climb the stairs to bed with hardly so much as a "hello." His tie would be loosened and his vest unbuttoned. I was becoming annoyed by his remoteness, yet I said nothing.

On Thursday evening he came home about 9:30. I had been alone for much of the day and really wanted to talk to him, but Ted had that glassy, faraway look in his eyes — a look I had come to know too well. Unwilling to face any other truth, I saw only his unwillingness to relate to me. I tried to start a conversation, but realized he wasn't even listening to me.

"You know, Ted," I said finally, "I'm getting pretty fed up. It seems to me that I have been giving, giving, giving to our relationship and I get virtually nothing in return—not even a few minutes' attention when I've hardly seen you all week."

Ted looked at me vaguely. "I'm really tired. I'm going up to bed."

"Why am I living with this man?" I asked myself. "I am getting absolutely nothing from this relationship." I was angry, frustrated, hurt, not only with the way I was being treated, but also with my own response. Why was I so hesitant to really confront him?

I returned home on Saturday from a brunch with friends to find Ted by the pool, beginning a spring cleanup. He was in a strangely foul mood. As he worked he flung a comment at me, "I've been out here thinking: What good is it to clean up this pool? It's a waste of effort." It didn't make sense to me at the time. Was he implying that we would not be living here to enjoy the pool? Or that *he* wouldn't? I was mystified, but his attitude was so vile that I couldn't respond. I joined him in the pool cleanup however, and as we worked very little was spoken by either of us. My silence spoke volumes about my fear of confrontation.

The next morning was Mother's Day. I can't remember going through the motions of gifts and a celebration with our four daughters, though we must have, for such observations were a firmly established tradition in our family. I do remember going to church, and that Ted declined to go with me.

I wasn't surprised; this was an increasingly frequent occurrence even though Ted had been very active in our congregation. Our church had always been a welcoming place, and we had many friends there. Now Ted seemed to withdraw from couples and groups of people whom we'd known for years — turning a cold shoulder and even ignoring them, especially when they were enjoying my companionship and conversation.

When I returned home that day he was sitting at the kitchen bar as if waiting for me to fix lunch. But when he looked at me the expression in his eyes sent a chill down my spine. To me it seemed the expression of a caged animal, raging with anger because it can't escape. Those intense blue eyes which had once conveyed so much warmth and laughter, so much love and joy, were now icy cold, and yet glaring with an emotion I could only interpret as hatred.

"There has to be more," he said, out of nowhere. "You don't give me what I need. Why aren't you what I want? What are we going to do about this situation? What are *you* going to do about it?"

I didn't know how to respond to this verbal onslaught. The void in our marriage was suddenly laid bare, and he was blaming me for being the root of the problem. I was overwhelmed, unable to organize my thoughts or words. Fear, guilt and confusion jammed my brain. The barriers I had erected between myself and reality were being attacked.

Ted wasn't interested in a response, however, and continued his attack. "I'm so attracted to energetic females," he said. "Why are you not energetic?"

Energetic? I thought about my weekly schedule, crammed full with work and volunteer commitments, family and home responsibilities, and social engagements. There was nothing wrong with my energy level! "What is this man talking about?" I thought.

"I like dark-haired, dark-eyed women," he said. "I find them intriguing." Ted's words inflicted another wound. Yet why should I defend my blonde hair and blue eyes or my English-Norwegian heritage?

"You never show any sparkle toward me," he said. "You light up whenever you see Joe or Sam or Paul, but you're never glad to see me. You would rather be with any other man than with me."

"That's not true," I protested, finally finding my voice. I needed to defend myself, however weakly.

"I don't know why you won't just admit that you'd rather be married to someone else," he said, "you don't have any feeling for me any more."

"That's not true," I repeated, "And there's no one else I want to be married to."

Ted did not seem to hear what I said.

"You just don't care a bit. It shows in the way you look at me and the way you act — never a bit of passion. I need passion in a woman," he snarled.

The hatred in his eyes was so intense that I was uncomfortable meeting his gaze. To calm myself, and to escape the emotional walls that were crashing down around me, I began preparing lunch. I needed something mundane, something familiar in this escalating situation. Ted stormed out to the patio to wait for me to serve the food. We ate a few bites in silence; then he began his accusations again.

"If you cared about me, you'd be glad to see me. But there's never any sign that you care. You really just don't give a damn any more, do you?"

"Ted, I *do* care," I protested. "I've asked that we spend more time together, and I've told you my concern about the lack of intimacy between us."

"No, you don't care." He wasn't trying to remember. He was determined that I was the source of all our problems. "You might as well admit it. You're happier when I'm not here. You're never glad to see me when I come home; you never show any delight when I come in."

My paralyzing confusion was subsiding and I began to state my case. "It's true that much of the sparkle *is* gone from our marriage, but I think it's gone on both sides. I feel that I have given a great deal to you and to the marriage and I've received very little in return. It's very hard for me to sparkle when I'm receiving no response from you. Sometimes I feel as though you aren't even present. You're physically present, but mentally and emotionally you're just not here."

"No, you don't care," Ted repeated. Again, he seemed not to have heard a word I said. "You'd rather be at church or at work or out gadding around instead of at home with me."

Ted was acting out as a naughty child would behave toward a parent, but he'd touched on a truth. I *had* learned to look for satisfaction outside our relationship.

My job was fulfilling; I enjoyed the work, and my colleagues were friendly and complimentary. My volunteer work with a local hospice made me feel needed and appreciated.

"I do receive a great deal of satisfaction from my job and my work at the hospice because people tell me they appreciate me. At home I never hear a word of thanks for any of my efforts."

"Maybe you care about the house and the kids," Ted admitted, "but you don't care about *me*. You never pay any attention to *me*."

I looked at him in amazement, remembering how much I had wanted to have an intimate conversation with him just a couple of evenings before. I also thought about all the times I had listened patiently to his long descriptions of problems at work, his feelings that people were "out to get" him. I had listened very carefully to his accounts, and had tried my best to understand them and help him deal with them.

"I *do* pay attention to you, Ted," I said simply.

"No, you don't care," he repeated. "You'd like to leave me; you know you would. Why don't you admit it?"

"I have thought of leaving," I said slowly, my denial ebbing. "I feel so few of my needs are being met in our relationship. The gap between us is like a chasm."

"I knew it!" he said triumphantly. "You've wanted to leave

for a long time. And you should have left. You should have left when I was out screwing around." The words hit me like a shot.

"You mean you have had other affairs since the one fifteen years ago, with Eleanor?" I asked tentatively, my breathing so shallow I felt it had ceased.

Ted didn't answer. He sat in silence with a kind of sneer on his face and nodded his head.

"You mean there have been other women?" I asked again.

This time he answered me. "Oh, yes."

My immediate response was feigned indifference. I couldn't let myself be hurt again; I couldn't let myself care.

I reached for a barrier to erect between myself and reality. "Well—so what?" I said bravely.

"And the reason is pretty simple," he said. "You just don't give me the things I need in a woman."

Suddenly I became aware that our teenage daughter, the youngest and only child still living at home, had entered the kitchen and was making herself a sandwich. I didn't want her to hear our conversation.

"Ted, if we are going to continue this discussion, I think we should go for a drive," I said.

"Fine with me," he answered. "It would be good to get out of here."

We drove out of town to a nearby park, wooded and lovely with its ponds and cascading water. I felt calmed by the beauty of our surroundings. But Ted was still raging about my inadequacies. He stopped the car near a high cliff.

"I need a woman who is vibrant and alive," he shouted. "You are so listless most of the time. I need a woman who is exciting. Since you don't give me what I need, of course I have looked for it elsewhere."

I fought to keep my defenses up, to keep from being hurt as badly as I had been by his first affair.

"There are lots of exciting women out there," he said,

"And I've simply gone out and found them." It was beginning to dawn on me that he was not talking about an occasional fling. I was stunned.

"Lots of them," he continued, somewhat incoherently. "Sometimes it's sickening how many there are. And sometimes I get sick of myself for screwing so many of them."

My expression must have conveyed my horror.

"I can't tell you how often I wanted to come home and confess what I was doing, " he said.

"Why didn't you?" I asked.

"I don't know. I thought you knew and just didn't care."

"I didn't know," I replied honestly.

"Sometimes I thought that the only way out was suicide," he continued. "I couldn't face the thought of your knowing."

Abruptly, he got out of our Pontiac. He walked to the edge of a waterfall and stood there, thrusting his hands deep into his pockets. I was numbed with the shock of Ted's revelation, but becoming conscious of a small sliver of pain. I looked at him, wondering if I should follow him. He might be thinking of throwing himself over the edge, solving his problems with dramatic finality; but in my shocked state I simply couldn't go to him. I had nothing left to give him, and a part of me didn't care if he jumped.

He returned to the car, utterly dejected: a man who couldn't go on, with nothing left to live for. He was oblivious to the pain that was washing over me. "Do you want out of the marriage?" I asked.

"No," he answered. "I'd like to see the marriage work. But you'll have to change." The conversation began moving in circles as he reiterated that I needed to be more exciting and "sparkling" so that he wouldn't have to find satisfaction elsewhere.

"I can tell that doing things for me is a great effort for you," he said. "It's as though I have become a terrible burden."

"I *have* felt a burden," I said, "because I feel that I have been giving beyond my capacity, and that I get very little in return."

"You know, you really don't understand the real world, Emma," he told me. "Everybody is out there screwing around."

"I know some people are," I acknowledged, "but I find it hard to believe that everyone is, or even that most people are. I think most people we know are faithful to their marriage vows."

"You'd be surprised," he said. "The whole world is doing it. You just don't understand about life in the fast lane."

"I guess I don't want to understand about it," I said.

Our conversation continued for hours, but only covered the same ground over and over again. The content included: How I wasn't meeting his needs, everyone was doing it and he had often wished to confess to me. I was incredulous when he said, "You are the one who needs to change in order to make our marriage work."

When we returned home I was exhausted, still in shock. Only after we had gone to bed and Ted was asleep did that small sliver of pain begin to throb, spreading throughout my whole being. I began sobbing, and Ted awoke. He looked at me, but didn't say anything.

"Could you just hold me?" I asked. He complied, but in the mechanical way that had become characteristic of our lovemaking. The full impact of what I was facing began to wash over me. I was devastated.

"I need my mother," I sobbed. "I want to talk to my mother." I desperately needed the security of her comfort and soothing touch. But talking to my mother was impossible; she had been dead for nine years.

Ted didn't respond. I was all alone.

Chapter I Exercise

Have there been times in your life when you have remained silent, even though you wanted to say something?

List three times you were silent.

1.

2.

3.

Have there been times that you were afraid to confront someone? List two times you were afraid.

1.

2.

Can you relate to any part of this story? Are there feelings coming up for you?

Write what those feelings are.

_____

_____

_____

_____

_____

_____

Notes

_____

_____

_____

_____

_____

_____

_____

_____

_____

_____

_____

_____

_____

_____

_____

_____

_____

_____

_____

_____

_____

_____

_____

_____

_____

_____

_____

_____

Chapter II

Testing the Secrets

"The Greek word for truth, aletha, means "not hidden""
- Catherine Kober

The weeks after that Mother's Day were painful as I learned more and more about Ted's secret life. I continued to ask him questions because I needed to admit a whole new dimension of Ted's personality. Questioning him about his life helped me face his reality.

"How soon after the first affair did the others start?" I asked, remembering back a dozen years.

"Right away," he told me.

"Had you wanted to have an affair before that?" I asked.

"Yes," he answered. "I had tried to set something up several times, but things didn't work out. I've been restless since the very beginning of our marriage. When we were first married, I used to make anonymous obscene phone calls to women I met at work."

Obscene phone calls! I couldn't believe what I was hearing. We were living in a small town at the time, and surely people would have recognized his voice! I expressed my shock. Ted shrugged.

The more we discussed it, the more I became aware that we had radically different ideas about sex and its relationship to love.

"Don't you ever want sex as a purely physical release?" he asked. "Don't you ever feel *driven* to have sex?"

"No," I answered. "Sex to me is a deep emotional expression of love. It's an important way to express love, but certainly not the only way."

Some of the difference in our attitudes toward sex could be seen as a difference commonly accepted in our culture, a difference between male and female views of sex. I knew that many men and women see sex, at least part of the time, as a purely physical release. Most of them are not sexual addicts. The key phrase was Ted's expression, *"driven* to have sex." He meant driven with an uncontrollable, absolutely irresistible force. Driven until he could think of nothing else but sexual satisfaction.

He talked about his fascination with women's clothing, the way it revealed the shape of the body underneath. He described watching women at the beach, comparing the difference in shapes of thighs and the configuration of the crotch, and how he found it difficult to think of anything else. Many men like to look at women, but Ted's focus on the subject was chilling, obsessive. He studied them as objects.

He told me how he would scrutinize a woman's posture, trying to decide if the way she stood meant an invitation for him to approach her. He said he wouldn't know until he made eye contact. After he caught a woman's eye he said, he could always tell whether or not she was willing.

Ted said he had considered going to prostitutes, but had never done it; why should he, when women were so easy to find, free of charge? He declared he could pick up a woman anywhere: at church, at the grocery store, at a party, and always at conventions. Such an encounter was especially promising at his telecommunications seminars and conventions — the relationship would last for the few days of the meeting, and often resume if both of them were at the next convention.

He confessed to becoming fascinated with having sex with a wide variety of physical types. He was determined to seduce one woman in particular because she was one of the most obese women he had ever met, even though he found obesity revolting.

Often women would ask, "Am I the only woman in your life besides your wife?" Invariably he would lie, "Of course." A big part of the thrill Ted got from his sexual encounters was the challenge of setting them up. Once he succeeded, much of the excitement was gone. The challenge of arranging the next rendezvous remained.

Another part of the challenge was devising reasons to get away—from me, from his family, from his work, always searching for new lies to tell. He told me about the time he spent planning sexual encounters and the amount of energy it took.

No wonder he had seemed tired so often!

Finally I became brave enough to ask him how many women he had taken to bed.

"Many," he answered.

I pushed.

"Are you talking about ten or fifteen?" I wanted to know. I thought knowing a number would help me understand, perhaps accept, what Ted had been telling me.

"More than that. I don't know how many. I suppose I could make a list."

Suddenly, I began making little connections in my head.

"Were you ever involved with _____ " I began naming names.

"You don't need me to make a list," he said. "You can make the list yourself."

"There are many that you know, but many more you don't know," he told me, "I have many ways of meeting them."

I looked at him. "Do you think that perhaps you are sick?" I asked.

"It has crossed my mind," he answered.

"Is it time for you to go for some help?"

"Maybe," he said.

Ted talked about "binging" on sex, a word significant for its association with addictions of all kinds, especially food and alcohol. He stated that he felt compelled to continue to find women, and he would keep dialing telephone numbers until he found someone available. He talked about the rush of excitement he felt when someone answered. It didn't matter *which* woman answered. If several contacts were made, he could sometimes arrange as many as three assignations in a day.

He said that sometimes after sex he would lie there and think, "Never again. This has got to stop." But no time was ever the last time and yes, he worried that his behavior was sick.

"When I found that I could go as long as three weeks without seeing someone, I figured I was okay," he said.

He saw some of the women in New York only two or three times; with others he had relationships that lasted for years, some ten years or more. All of these "relationships" were based on physical contact. Ted described how he would call a woman, meet her briefly for sex, and leave immediately afterward. Many times he planned a work-related appointment so that he would have an excuse to leave. "I didn't want to talk to them," he explained.

"Things had to become more and more perverted in order to be interesting," he said. "I want to tell you how perverted some of it was." But I had heard all I wanted to hear for the time being.

I had heard enough to know that what he was telling me was real, and I no longer wanted to hear more details because it sounded so sick. I was becoming so nauseated I was afraid

I was going to vomit. It felt as though he was purging himself of all his guilt, lies and betrayal and I was the container to hold the bitter bile.

I thought back over the past few years, seeing other signs of Ted's sexual addiction. I had occasionally come into our bedroom to discover him staring out the window.

"What are you staring at?" I asked.

"Oh, nothing," he would say. In retrospect, it occurred to me that he was looking into the bathroom of the house next door. The family included two teenaged daughters who were often careless about pulling the blind. I realized he watched them shower and dress.

As far as I knew, however, Ted's "peeping Tom" behavior never extended beyond our bedroom window. Nor did he engage in exhibitionism or other aberrant behaviors that sexual addicts sometimes adopt. I don't believe that he was excessively involved with pornography, frequently an obsession with the sexual addict. I actually don't know, however; I never learned what he meant by "really perverted" behavior.

More devastating to me was Ted's attitude toward his secret life and his attitude toward me. In spite of reporting having felt a kind of remorse, and vowing "never again," he did not apologize to me. He never addressed or acknowledged the searing pain he caused me, the unraveling effect his behavior was having on my life.

He had been conscious of hurting me at the time of his first affair, and said, "I never want to hurt you like this again." I found some comfort then, in his responsiveness to my feelings. The revelations were so much more overwhelming and Ted seemed oblivious that he was hurting me so deeply. I began to understand this as a sign of the progress of his illness from reading Patrick Carnes', *Out of the Shadows* book.

As the days passed, I realized I could no longer hide the ugliness that had entered our lives. The burden of carrying

Ted's secret was too much for me. I went to the office of a friend, Jack Overmeyer, who had worked with us in some business ventures, ostensibly for the purpose of discussing financial matters.

As I sat down, he said with great concern, "Emma, you look awful. You look absolutely beaten. What's going on?" He stood up and walked over to close the office door.

I took a deep breath and told him of Ted's revelations and how devastated I felt. His response was supportive, but surprising.

"I'm so glad you finally confided in me," he said. "We've known for a long time that something was wrong, and we've been concerned."

Slowly and cautiously I began to tell him some of the details of Ted's life. I wasn't certain how much he wanted to hear, and I was so distraught that I wasn't capable of telling him much. It was enough, though, to open the floodgates on my feelings. When I left shortly thereafter and went back to my own office, I called Ted.

"I'm coming over to see you," I said. "I'll be there in twenty minutes."

I reached his small, tidy office, which appeared larger because of a window at one end. I marched straight in and made my announcement. "I'm going to start seeing a psychiatrist," I said. "And I'm also going to contact a divorce lawyer."

At these words Ted looked frightened.

"I don't care what *you* do," I said, "But these are the steps I'm going to take. I would hope that you would get some help." At that point I didn't know whether I wanted to stay with him or not. Much depended on his response and behavior.

True to my word, I took both of my announced steps. First, I found a lawyer and got her advice regarding my rights and my financial situation. She listened to my story with much sympathy and shook her head. "A man like that will never change," she said.

The other professional I consulted was a highly recommended psychiatrist. He, too, listened to my story empathetically. His prognosis for my marriage was only slightly more optimistic; he gave it a five percent chance for improvement. "Out of a hundred men who have this problem, perhaps five will change their behavior," he said.

I wanted to believe that Ted could be one of the five percent; I wanted to believe that he could change. So I was delighted when he found Jungian analyst Helen Smith somewhere else in the city and started therapy. Leaving directly from work for his late afternoon appointments, Ted was always dressed impeccably in three-piece suits and silk ties. It was important to him to look like the telecommunications professional that he was. I imagine it was also very difficult for him to take the step of seeing a therapist.

On Ted's second or third visit to the therapist, she suggested he may have a sexual addiction, and mentioned that it might be helpful for him to read *Out of the Shadows*. He stormed out of her office in the middle of the session, outraged and refusing to consider that he had a serious addiction. He came home and told me what his therapist had said. "Yes," I thought to myself. "It's true."

According to experts in the field of addictions, an addict will rarely admit a problem until a crisis forces a recognition. I discovered that I had precipitated such a crisis for Ted by seeking help for myself. Ted now knew that I was serious about making changes in our lives, and he was frightened that I would leave him. "What will you do if the therapist tells you to leave?" he asked me. Following his exploration of the symptoms described in the book and after several days of consideration, Ted admitted that he was, indeed, a sexual addict.

"Do you want to change?" I asked Ted.

"Yes," he said, "I do."

He had taken the first step. Since we now both acknowledged the ugly secret in our lives, we might be able to work together to rid ourselves of it.

When Ted next went to his analyst, she asked if I would be willing to join their therapy sessions. I agreed. I wanted to heal my own wounds and to discover what my role had been in the drama. I wanted to assist his recovery and to mend our marriage, making it meaningful again for both of us. Thus for a period of about six months I was involved in therapy sessions twice a week — once to see my own therapist and once to work with Ted and his therapist.

As I look back on this period, it occurs to me that our treatment was not adequate. The addicted partner was receiving less intense therapy, only once a week in sessions attended by his spouse, while the spouse was receiving in-depth therapy in private sessions with a psychiatrist in addition to the joint sessions. Now I wonder whether Ted could have been helped more if he had received in-depth private therapy, perhaps one or two private sessions weekly. Ted's choice of a therapist was excellent. She was sincerely interested in helping him change as she involved me in the process. In the sessions she established an atmosphere in which Ted and I could be more open and honest with each other than we had been since the early days of our marriage.

In the beginning I had high hopes for the success of our therapies. Ted focused on the process with great energy and cooperated fully with Helen, the therapist. She requested that he apologize to the women with whom he had affairs. Ted complied to some extent. I saw a letter he wrote to one woman who lived out of the state, and knew that he called at least five others to say, "It's over." It appeared he was making a concerted effort to change his life.

The therapist next asked Ted to apologize to his family, and once again he complied. He met with all four of our daughters, apologizing for his behavior. It did not make amends for the hurt he had inflicted on them, which was much too deep to be cured by an apology, but it was a first gesture.

Finally, the therapist asked Ted if he thought his behavior had affected his performance as an executive or if his co-workers had been hurt by it. Ted admitted he supposed his secretary and assistant had both at least been inconvenienced by what he had done. Again he was asked to apologize, but he never complied.

Ted was unable to act upon another suggestion made by the therapist. She advised that the best type of therapy for his problem would be a sexual addiction group based on the principles of Alcoholics Anonymous (AA). Such a group did not yet exist in our area, so she recommended he join a white collar AA group. While Ted said he'd think about it, he never joined, apparently unable to reveal his secret to a support group.

During this period of a few months, Ted appeared to be aware of both our needs in the marriage, understanding what we both had to give to make the marriage work. He seemed to desire, as much as I did, the honesty, openness and commitment that could make our marriage fulfilling again for both of us.

"I am so glad you are staying with me through this," he told me over and over. His therapist later told me that, in his first session, Ted had broken down and sobbed, utterly distraught with the fear that I would leave him. She assigned us several books to read together. One, *Invisible Partners*, by John Sanford, is a book describing the "animus" and the "anima" of Jungian psychology, and how these principles affect each individual. Ted was fascinated, and we had several intense, highly satisfying discussions about the book and how its theories applied to us. The sharing and intimacy we achieved in these discussions was unlike anything we had experienced for years. I truly felt we were making marvelous progress.

By the end of the summer, however, I began to have doubts. I realized that I was very angry about his behavior all those years. I felt a great need to express my fury and have him recognize the tremendous hurt that was causing it. Ted couldn't deal with my anger. At my slightest expression of anger, he would withdraw into silence. It seemed to me as if he had crawled into a shell for protection or to hide from the situation.

"We aren't going to make it, are we?" he would say.

"Yes, we can make it," I said, "But we need to express all of our feelings." But Ted didn't want to recognize negative feelings. He saw me as his "angry mother." He didn't want to admit his own rage, which he projected onto me.

Finally, my own rage erupted. Never in my life have I felt so out of control as I did on the day of that emergency session with the therapist. All day I had been pacing and crying constantly, vacillating between tears of anguish and tears of rage. My emotions were coming out, but I was frightened of my loss of control. I had thoughts and feelings of wanting to hurt myself or someone else. This episode made Ted retreat from me into a silent fear.

The silence was devastating after the intimate, meaningful discussions we had shared so recently. Yet I knew the "Jekyll and Hyde" behavior is characteristic of addicts of all kinds. One minute the adult is in charge and the addict wants to make a change, but soon the uncontrollable child takes charge, resulting in emotional pain that can lead back to the addictive behavior.

I was stymied. I knew that dealing with anger is a crucial aspect of any relationship, that we had to learn what to do with our wrath. We were encouraged to continue to talk about our anger, but Ted did not want to cooperate.

In September I planned a church retreat at a lodge in the Adirondacks. Based on our discussions in therapy about my need for positive feedback from Ted, I asked him to provide affirmation for me while I was away. I asked him to make a list about all the things he liked about me, to be given to me on my return. When I returned, however, he had forgotten. I reminded him, and he angrily scribbled a couple of words on a tiny piece of scrap paper. I felt as though I had been slapped.

Shortly thereafter we left for a long-planned trip to Europe. I savored the tastes of new-found wines along the Rhine and the beauty of the Black Forest in Germany. While we sat in a meadow with a picnic lunch in the Swiss Alps, I was sure Julie Andrews would come over the hill singing "The Sound of Music." Beautiful pastoral scenes were accented by the ringing of cowbells. In Budapest we were treated to a memorable opera, but the only color in Czechoslovakia was the red star on the gray buildings. It was such a contrast to the flowerboxes studding the neat white German houses. I was glad that Ted was agreeable to all of my suggestions for sightseeing and activities, but I sensed that he wasn't enjoying himself. It seemed the trip was a duty for him. He tried to shorten our trip from six weeks to four, so that he could attend a conference. I later learned that his plan was to meet a woman there.

Several weeks after our trip I asked Ted about a colleague of his who had been seriously ill.

"He's become worse since we visited him," Ted responded.

"We?" I asked.

When I pressed him, he admitted that, during the September weekend I was out of town, he had visited the hospital with a female colleague, whom he then took out to dinner. She was the reason he had forgotten to make the list I had requested. The deception was beginning again, and I was indignant. He continued to be afraid of my anger, barring me from expressing it. As Sanford described in *Invisible Partners*, Ted's fear was causing him to resort to childish reactions.

By Christmas, as I tried to go about all the holiday activities of shopping, wrapping and baking our family's favorite treats, I felt stung by the certainty that therapy was not helping. The chasm between us seemed as wide as ever. We had been in therapy about six months, a time period I later learned is significant. Patrick Carnes, one of the most prominent experts on sexual addiction, says that six months is a critical period for the sexual addict who is trying to change his behavior. He states that after six months many, many addicts give up their efforts to change, slipping back into their addiction, often permanently. Ted was proving to be a textbook case.

Many households suffer increased stress during holiday periods, and our relationship reached a crisis point just before Christmas. Ted told me on the morning of Christmas Eve that he had decided to move out.

"Go ahead and go," I said. "If you think that I really don't care about you, go ahead and go."

Relatives and friends were coming for dinner that evening, but I was not going to put up a front any longer. I would serve the meal myself and tell the truth about Ted's absence. I was finished with keeping secrets.

He stomped around the house for several hours and then came back to tell me he had changed his mind.

"I'm thinking more clearly," he said, "I know you do care for me."

Later in therapy we discussed what was missing in our marriage for both of us — intimacy, a sense of connectedness and caring. But our relationship did not improve.

"I wish Emma were more supportive," he said, "I wish she would meet me at the door when I come home in the evenings." For the next few days I made a point of being at the door when he arrived home after work. He sidestepped my embrace and wouldn't look at me.

"Emma is following through on everything I ask," he conceded in therapy, "But I have no feelings for her. It does nothing for me when she walks into the room."

I was incredulous. I screamed in anger, "How can you say that, when I have stood by you for the last nine months, trying so hard to understand, being supportive and making changes you have requested?"

My spirit had been crushed one more time, and I moved one step closer to the realization that this relationship was disintegrating — one step closer to ending my denial.

Privately, I told the therapist, "He is no longer working on his problem."

"Is he having another affair?" she asked.

"No, I don't think so," I answered.

I was wrong.

I learned the truth in March when he returned from another business trip to Chicago. When I met him at the plane, he was "too tired" to talk, and he made love to me in a mechanical, meaningless way. He had no interest in intimacy or sharing of any kind, and his eyes had the haunted look of someone who isn't really present.

Shortly after his return, I found out that the woman he had taken to dinner during my absence in September had been his constant companion during his business trip. I concluded he had been deceiving me with her for the last six months, while he continued to go through the motions of therapy with me.

Suddenly, it dawned on me that Ted was never going to change. If I continued to adapt for him, I soon would be a walking, emotionless shell, with his fantasy world rolling over me, crushing me as it was destroying him. My denial about his behavior, about my own pain and trauma was beginning to wane, but it was not over.

Learning the truth of his latest affair, I screamed with rage. He regarded me with the expression of a small boy being chastised by his mother. Now I knew I would never have an adult, mature relationship with this man. No matter how much I gave, it would never be enough.

Another piece of the truth was confirmed in April. During Holy Week, Ted and I often went to the Maundy Thursday service together. As the Passion story was read and the candles extinguished, congregants left the sanctuary in silence, awaiting Easter Sunday. This particular time, I went to the service alone, which had lately become my routine. As I left the church, I had no idea that Ted was developing a plan that closed the door on any possible reconciliation.

When I returned home, Ted was occupied at the game table, constructing a budget. However, this budget was not the usual family financial statement. This one was really two; one for each of us. At this point, I realized that a true reconciliation would not be in our future. While I had been working on salvaging our marriage, Ted had been working on demolishing it. The darkness of Maundy Thursday was echoed by the darkness of our home.

Had I wasted the year in therapy with Ted? I don't think so. It was a year of revealed secrets, explored solutions and struggles to understand him. I was able at last to talk openly about my feelings. It ended with the satisfaction of knowing that I had done everything I could to make the marriage work. Ted's therapist supported my conclusion.

Oddly enough, we continued to do things together, like any other couple. Five days before he moved out, we went to the theater. The play was the story of country singer G.W. Lincoln's life, and his struggle with alcoholism. G.A. Lincoln, too, had lost relationships. Ultimately he lost his life. I held Ted's hand through the play, squeezing it when we heard poignant lines and songs from the stage. He did not respond.

Ted moved out in May. He said he had to leave to keep his

sanity. He had decided that his problem could be solved by leaving me and living with another woman. She had told him that her love could make him a different person, and he continued to believe that his happiness lay somewhere outside himself, rejecting the need for inner change.

This time I didn't hesitate. I contacted several friends who had gone through divorces, asking for opinions or recommendations of lawyers they had employed. I received eight attorneys' names, chose three to interview, two women and one man, and found the one I felt to be the best person to represent me. I made my selection carefully. The male attorney seemed depressed and not very interested in my case. The first female attorney I visited was so aggressive she was filling out papers and telling me what my settlement would look like before my information interview was over. I settled on the third person, a woman who patiently explained the process to me and at the end of our conversation asked, "What do you want to do?"

It was time for me to take control of my own life and choose its direction. At long last I acknowledged the ugly secrets in my life; I had made a good faith effort at resolving them and now I was moving to rid myself of their oppression.

Chapter II Exercise

Has there been a time when you have felt rage and out of control?

List three times you were out of control.
1.

2.

3.

What were the situations that made you have those feelings?
1.

2.

3.

Write about your feelings.

_____
_____
_____
_____
_____
_____

Chapter II Exercises continued

Do you feel as though you are struggling to keep your relationship together? How are you trying to keep it together? Write about the things you are doing to keep the relationship?

_____

_____

_____

_____

_____

_____

_____

_____

_____

_____

_____

_____

_____

_____

_____

_____

_____

_____

_____

_____

_____

_____

_____

_____

_____

_____

_____

_____

_____

Notes

_____
_____
_____
_____
_____
_____
_____
_____
_____
_____
_____
_____
_____
_____
_____
_____
_____
_____
_____
_____
_____
_____
_____
_____
_____
_____
_____

Chapter III

The Secrets Begin

"Like an ability or a muscle, hearing your inner wisdom is strengthened by doing it" — *Robbie Grass*

"What I am actually saying is that we need to be willing to let our intuition guide us, and then be willing to follow that guidance directly and fearlessly." — *Shakti Gawain*

"This world needs more couples like you two will be," the letter said. It was a letter of congratulations from our high school English teacher, Mary Samantha MacArthur, written after she had seen the announcement of our engagement in our hometown newspaper. Many people shared her feelings, and I felt very lucky. I firmly believed for fifteen years that I was fortunate to have a wonderful husband and a rock-solid marriage.

I had known Ted literally all my life. I cannot remember where or when I first saw him — in a small town everyone knows everyone else. Our paths crossed frequently in childhood, even though we attended different elementary schools. As a young girl I wasn't interested in Ted; even as a young teenager I wasn't attracted to him. By the time we were upperclassmen we were dating, however, and I was proud to be seen with him. We went on to Cornell University, and decided to get married after my sophomore year, his junior year.

Everyone who knew us was pleased. His grandmother said, "As long as you two have been together, you must have been meant for each other."

We were truly in love in those days. I can remember how our first apartment rang with laughter, as we enjoyed each other's company. Ted belonged to several organizations at the time, including his college fraternity, but he would sometimes forgo those obligations to be with me. In those days we could talk for hours—I thought we would never run out of things to say. Our sex life was healthy and mutually satisfying, and I saw its pleasures as a symbol of our love and commitment.

Our first three daughters were born within the first six years of our marriage, and Ted was interested and involved in my pregnancies and participating with the new arrivals. His involvement was remarkable for a man of the times, just before the 1960's and the women's movement.

Because money was tight, we became adept at finding inexpensive yet enjoyable means of recreation. We especially enjoyed games, from Monopoly to tennis, taking mutual delight in the competition, and involved the children as they grew older.

Our recreational circle included other young couples with children. Activities were organized around potluck suppers and bridge, usually with the children in attendance. Ted and I discovered that we were good Bridge partners, communicating well.

Camping was an enjoyable form of recreation we could afford. Our camping trips offered a means of learning new things—about the natural world and new places. We introduced the children to nature.

Gardening was a hobby we both embraced. We planned our vegetable and flower gardens with attention to plants that would grow well together and thrive in our local area. Ted grew his favorites, focusing on the vegetable garden, especially tomatoes. He enjoyed making early season gifts of homegrown tomatoes to surprised friends and neighbors. My interest was the flowers, from crocus in the early spring to asters and chrysanthemums in the late fall. We both delighted in the beauty and productivity of our garden.

Our sense of commitment to our own future and family extended to our community from our earliest years together. We had many friends. Ted belonged to several civic organizations, and we were active members of our church. I belonged to a sisterhood dedicated to improving education for women.

One reason we were able to make friends so easily was that Ted was gregarious and charming. He never had a problem walking into a room full of strangers — they didn't remain strangers for long. People were delighted by his open, friendly manner, and they talked easily with him almost immediately. I have since realized that Ted's relationships, although quickly formed, were almost always lacking in depth, matching the clinical description of the relationships of an addict. It appeared to me that his interaction with others remained superficial, invariably revolving around sports or the latest bad snowstorm. His conversations with friends and acquaintances never reached the level of shared feelings, hopes and life priorities. At the time, however, I could only envy the ease with which he made new friends. I was the quiet one, following his lead, but discovering my own new friends as well.

Time passed, and our lives continued to change for the better. We moved to New Rochelle, a suburb closer to Ted's company. The Presbyterian Church there was a great place for Ted to volunteer his leadership skills. He freely gave many hours of his time to serve as chair for numerous committees. Interviewing and hiring new personnel was second nature to him because, as an executive in his company he was doing it constantly. Even though Ted had no training in the area of education, he had an interest in the education programs at the church. He volunteered to get some training to be a lay leader in some of the religious education classes for adults. He was able to facilitate lively, thought-provoking discussion in the groups.

We made new friends. We discovered do-it-yourself skills in each of us as we decorated and landscaped first our new home and then a cabin in a mountain area a short drive from the city.

During these times Ted and I worked well together and arguments were rare. Looking back, I realize that all this "busy-ness" kept our focus on external things. We were absorbed with doing and accomplishing and filling our lives with social relationships. We were so busy we didn't take time to focus on developing an intimate relationship. Although we were working together much of the time, we were so involved in our projects we actually created a distance from one another. At the time I felt proud of the work we did together. I saw it as evidence of the effectiveness of our marriage. Only in hindsight do I see the rift that slowly was developing between us. We shared work; we shared activities and interests; but we did not share what was in our hearts.

As time went on we had more time for our community involvement. We both assumed positions of leadership in our church. I taught Sunday school while he held a series of positions, which led to his becoming clerk of Session. Ted joined a civic organization in our New Rochelle suburb and I joined a chapter of Women for Continuing Education (WCE).

In the corporate arena Ted was an organization whiz. He had the ability to oversee and manage many projects at the same time. As his secretary stated, "I have never known anyone who could juggle so many things at one time." Much of his time was spent in required meetings. In the brief periods of uninterrupted time, Ted could swiftly make decisions concerning messages and items on his agenda that needed immediate attention. Colleagues and employees respected his prompt responsiveness to urgent business matters. At a company holiday party, Matthew, who was head of sales, said to me, "I am so grateful Ted is at the helm, because he is a clear and organized thinker."

During this time Ted also became interested in the problem of drug use among young people, rampant in many parts of the U.S. in the mid-sixties. He joined a group which worked to help young people with drug problems. He came home with wrenching tales about young people who ran away from home and starved themselves in order to buy drugs. Eventually, we became involved with the teenage drug problem in a very personal way, taking in a fourteen-year-old girl who was ineligible for community shelter programs. I became very fond of her, glad that we had been able to help her, and proud that our marriage was strong enough that we could reach out to a young person in such a special way.

Everything about our lives seemed to go smoothly in those years following our move. Our three daughters were in school, and I was thinking about returning to work full-time when I discovered I was pregnant with our fourth daughter. Although I was disappointed that I was going to have to put my career on hold a few more years, I was delighted with the baby. It seemed a turning point, however, in my relationship with Ted. His lack of empathy at my having to change my plans made me begin to realize that he had never been particularly supportive of my efforts to make a career for myself.

After I learned of Ted's addiction, I was fascinated to read of the link between some personality disorders and addiction, particularly sexual addiction. These personality disorders involve a preoccupation with one's own fantasies, wishes and needs, a lack of empathy for others and a desire to control and dominate others rather than to engage in mutual relationships. Many sexual addicts seem to meet these diagnostic criteria, but during these early years I couldn't even see the personality disorders, much less the sexual addiction.

Apparently, however, the sexual addiction was present even during the happier years. Much, much later Ted told me that before we moved from our hometown he had indulged in behavior that Carnes (author of the book *Out of the Shadows)* would probably classify as Level II sexual addictive activity. Among the activities of Level II addiction is indecent phone calls. Other activities include exhibitionism, voyeurism and indecent liberties, such as inappropriate touching. Even now, as I think very carefully over that time, I recall no overt sign of deviant sexual behavior or attitude. Ted kept his secret well without leaving a clue.

Overlooking Ted's occasional selfishness, I was happy during those early years. I was in love with him and proud of the fact that he was my husband. I believed our marriage was built on commitment and communication, a foundation that would keep it intact no matter what challenges life brought us.

It all began to change just before our fifteenth wedding anniversary. Ted had started graduate school at New York University. Much later I was interested to read in Carnes' *Out of the Shadows,* that graduate school or other high-stress situations often serve as a catalyst for the emergence of sexual addiction. The addict escapes from his or her daily stresses by withdrawing into a secret world of fantasy or by having a sexual "fix." The addict substitutes external sources of self-soothing for his or her undeveloped internal resources. Addicts seek a mood-altering chemical or behavior in order to change an unpleasant emotion caused by the stress.

Ted had been out of town for a week, attending a convention in conjunction with his graduate studies. When I met him at Newark Airport, I immediately sensed something strange. He was exuberantly glad to see me, and as soon as he entered the airport he swept me up in a big bear hug, kissing me enthusiastically. Although we had been physically playful at home, he had never before been so physical after his return from a trip. I felt his enthusiasm was not genuine. There was giddiness about his behavior, an unusual amount of light-hearted laughter. "He's never acted this way before," I said to myself. I noticed that he was wearing a tie I had never seen.

"Oh, you bought a new tie while you were there," I said. No, he assured me, he had not purchased the tie. It had been a gift. While he was attending the convention he had organized a fishing trip for a group of guys. They had bought him the tie as a token of their appreciation for his efforts. I had no reason to question his explanation; it sounded plausible enough at the time.

A couple of hours later we met some good friends for a welcome home dinner. Ted seemed his usual jovial self, and we had a nice evening. I noticed nothing strange or unusual in his behavior at dinner.

After we returned home, however, his behavior again seemed different. I was eager to make love, but for the first time in our marriage, Ted was not responsive. He didn't at all act like a man who had been away from his wife for a week. Finally, very late in the evening, we did have sex, but his actions seemed forced. I felt as though he really wasn't present. In fifteen years of marriage, he never acted that way and I was mystified.

A week later was our fifteenth anniversary and we arranged for a baby-sitter so that we could celebrate at our special retreat, our wilderness cabin. The weekend lacked an air of celebration from the very beginning. Ted talked some about the convention he had attended, in particular about an impressive woman he had met from the Boston area. He told me many details about her job, her husband, her children and her life. I wondered how he had a chance to spend so much time talking with her.

As the weekend progressed, Ted grew more and more remote. I became extremely frustrated because, no matter what I did, I couldn't seem to connect with him. He was preoccupied and spacey, and his behavior was maddening to me. Finally, when we went for a walk together in the woods, I confronted him.

"What is going on?" I blurted, "You have changed, and I can't reach you. Is there another woman?" I hadn't realized that I suspected such a thing until the words were out of my mouth.

He readily admitted it. She was the woman he had talked about with such enthusiasm. He had met her the first afternoon of his Miami conference. They were in bed within two hours. He labeled it "love at first sight." She was thrilled with his attention. Never before had he known such lovemaking, and he went on to describe their passionate sex in vivid detail. He said he couldn't respond to me the first night after he came home because he was afraid he would utter her name instead of mine.

"That tie didn't come from a group of fishermen," I stammered in a daze.

He confessed. The tie had been a present from her.

My first reaction was, "What's wrong with me?" I knew that I had been a good wife. I thought that our sex life had been mutually satisfying. Why would Ted need an affair? The hurt I felt was overwhelming and I sobbed uncontrollably. I wanted Ted to talk to me, to tell me why he had done it. He was glad to comply.

"I've always wanted that kind of experience," he said, "Where you meet someone and know instantly that you belong together. I've always known that the sex would be marvelous with that kind of attraction." He said he had tried before to find a situation in which there was instant attraction and then instant, wonderful sex, but he had always failed. He had felt attractions before, but the sex had never followed.

Years later, I began to realize that sexual activity can be and frequently is equated with love and acceptability. Sex is sought as a nurturing agent. At the time I could only ask myself again, "What's wrong with me?" I heard a little answer in the back of my mind, "Nothing. Nothing is wrong with you." I wanted to know that the little voice was speaking the truth.

"Don't you realize how much you are hurting me?" I asked, "Why would you do such a thing?"

"I guess I thought I deserved someone better than you," he said bluntly.

How difficult it was to cling to the wisdom of that little voice in my head!

"Maybe I'm at fault fifty percent," I said, "But I don't think I am. And I will never take more than fifty percent of the blame for this." I burst into tears of grief and rage.

"Please don't be so upset, Emma," he said, "And please don't do anything to hurt yourself. Stay away from the edge of the cliff."

The thought of hurting myself had not entered my mind, and I had not noticed that we were near the edge of a cliff. But the tears wouldn't stop flowing, no matter how much I tried to control them. Ted wanted to comfort me, but the only way he could think of to comfort me was to have sex. That wasn't the comfort I wanted.

We returned home in silence; I was conscious of nothing but a heavy numbness. I felt I was drowning in choked-up emotions of all kinds.

When we reached the house I found the necktie, chopped it into little tiny pieces and burned them in the fireplace. The anger I felt toward this unknown woman consumed me. I continued to misdirect my anger, aiming it at her rather than at the person closest to me. I desperately wanted to believe she had initiated the affair; then I could explain away my husband's behavior. Toward Ted I felt only disbelief and hurt.

Ted was convinced that, after knowing this woman for five days, he was passionately in love with her. He was ready to marry her. He wrote her a long letter, saying that he was moving to her town. She responded immediately, calling him at work to tell him she was married. She had no intention of leaving her husband, she hardly knew Ted and the affair was over. Ted came home and told me of the phone call.

"I will never have another affair," he told me, "because I never want to hurt you like this again." I wanted desperately to believe that he was telling the truth. Our life had seemed so good. How could this happen?

At the time I was so torn apart I did not recognize how bizarre this infidelity had been. No, this was not a one-night stand, an indiscretion brought on by alcohol. No, this was not a long friendship that had gone over the boundaries into intimacy. This was a five-day sexual frenzy with a stranger. Now he wanted to leave his wife, his family and his job, move to another town, marry the stranger and live happily ever after!

I began to question the quality of our intimacy and, certainly, Ted's commitment to the relationship. Was I so horribly duped, or had I colluded in projecting this "perfect" marriage in our world?

I knew we needed some good marriage counseling. I begged Ted to go with me. He refused. He said he had made a mistake but that it would never happen again and we had no need for counseling. I considered going to counseling alone, but couldn't find the courage. How I wish someone had talked with me then and helped me summon the courage to discover how beneficial counseling could be.

Living with the secret of Ted's infidelity was very difficult. I thought about confiding in close friends, but I was ashamed. I was stung by the idea that if I told anyone, even a very close friend, she would know that I had been rejected by my husband.

At last, I felt I couldn't stand the pain any longer and talked with two close friends. Both listened sympathetically and neither expressed any form of censure toward me. One of the women, Maria Brick, was the one who had joined us for dinner after Ted's return from the convention.

"I thought Ted was behaving strangely that evening," she said.

"Why?" I asked.

She thought carefully. "His gaiety seemed forced," she said, "And he wouldn't look me in the eye. He usually does."

I thought back over that evening. I could not remember any of the behavior she described, but certainly had noticed something wrong when we reached home.

I found great relief in talking with my friends and was sorry that I had waited so long to confide. I also talked at great length with Ted. He was contrite, now that the affair was over.

"I made a mistake," he said, "And I'm sorry. I promise you I'll never be sexually involved with anyone else again." He appeared so sincere that I couldn't help but believe him. But believing him was probably easier than it should have been because I wanted so desperately to believe.

Later I learned that addicts experience a cyclical pattern of altered mood and behavior that is relatively impervious to conscious control. Environmental or internal stimuli triggers sexual fantasies that develop into a compelling craving to carry out the fantasized act. A trance-like excitement builds, heightened by risk and danger as, the plan develops for the next sexual encounter. An intense "high" during anticipation and completion of the act may be followed by fear, disgust, depression and remorse, coupled with a short-lived resolve never to repeat the act. I saw this pattern for the first time in Ted's reactions to his affair. Fortunately for my peace of mind at the moment, I didn't know it was a pattern. Nor did I understand that residual discomfort is relieved by increasing preoccupation with new sexual fantasies and thus the cycle repeats.

These cycles inflicted emotional abuse on me. Ted's moods were not predictable, and I was constantly on edge, trying to do everything in my power to prevent a bad mood.

I did realize that bonds had been broken. I struggled to regain trust in his commitment to the relationship, but it was impossible to have the same level of trust. On an intuitive level, it did not seem he was working on the relationship. I had the same feeling as I do in a conversation when someone is not listening. I had lost respect for him because he was not the person he claimed to be.

I tried to pretend that our lovemaking was as good as ever, but Ted never was truly present when we made love after that. For me, our bed now had a third person in it—the other woman. My mind constantly asked: "Am I being compared to her or to whomever he is really thinking about right now?" Much later I learned that he was involved in new affairs within weeks of his passionate declarations of fidelity, true to the pattern of the sexual addict.

We were to live with these secret affairs for a dozen years to come. They dominated our lives. We never mentioned them. On a conscious level, I did not acknowledge them, but a large part of our energy was devoted to keeping them secret. These secrets corrupted our life, and we let them do so. His behavior caused me to be "off balance" about what was real or unreal and what was the truth or a lie. My behavior allowed it to continue. He would deny statements he had made the previous day. I thought I was going crazy. Over the years I slid into a black hole of depression. By the twenty-seventh year of our marriage the depression was severe.

Chapter III Exercise

Have you given up being true to yourself? When were you free to express who you really are? Do a little sleuth work in order to restore the person you have abandoned; yourself. You may feel strong emotions as you retrieve memories.

1) How have I given up being true to myself?

_____

_____

_____

_____

_____

2) In what ways do I not trust myself?

_____

_____

_____

_____

_____

3) What did I used to do that I don't do anymore, but wish I still did?

_____

_____

_____

_____

_____

Notes

Chapter IV

The Secrets I Kept
From Myself

"Every time you don't follow your inner guidance, you feel a loss of energy, loss of power, a sense of spiritual deadness."
- Sahkti Gawain

"You will know the truth and the truth will set you free."
- John 8:32

On our fifteenth wedding anniversary I confronted Ted about my suspicion that he was having an affair, but for the next dozen years of our marriage I lived in denial that he was having more affairs. Though all the symptoms were obvious, the defense mechanism of denial allowed me to refuse to accept important aspects of reality. Denial kept me from contemplating the possibility that Ted was having another affair—a possibility that was too painful for me to face. I repeatedly distorted reality to fit my denial, but that denial left me exposed to a great deal of emotional abuse.

My behavior was typical in a relationship with an addict. An alcoholic, drug addict or compulsive gambler will attempt to hide and deny his or her obsession from their spouse or lover, and the loved one will collude in the destructive behavior. Ted encouraged my denial because he, too, did not want to admit to or deal with his addiction. Thus "supported" by Ted, I felt justified in hiding from the truth about the menace in our lives. My denial delayed our confronting the problem and the chaos and trauma it would create. What might happen to our marriage, family life, security of home? I also had concerns about Ted's mental stability: would he do something to harm himself or his family?

Until very recently, society's attitude toward addiction of any kind has presented a tremendous obstacle to recognizing the problem. In the past, addiction has been seen as a character and moral flaw rather than an illness, and no one wanted to admit that a loved one was so tainted. By removing the veil of denial I would have to admit to family and friends that there was a serious problem in our house. I wanted everyone, including myself, to believe that ours was the perfect family.

Society's censure of addiction has been slow to lift, and even now admission of addiction often results in condemnation, which increases the difficulty in dealing with the problem. Because sex addiction has only recently been recognized as an addictive behavior, society is even less inclined to be understanding of this problem than of other addictions. It is not acceptable to be an alcoholic, but it is acceptable to be sexual, even in an unhealthy way, because we are sexual beings. Our society bombards us with reminders of sexuality—on the television, billboards, movies, magazines and books. The "cool" behavior for men is to be "sexual Machos," while women are to be the objects.

So I stood between Ted, the addict, and the crisis of exposing his behavior. I was enabling and condoning his continuation of our dilemma. Was I beginning to display some symptoms of his illness?

I believed Ted when he said that first affair was over, and he may have been sincere in his initial resolve not to hurt me, to be a faithful husband. Yet the parade of women through his life began very soon after his passionate pledge of fidelity. He betrayed me terribly, of course, but there is a sense in which I betrayed myself.

As Ted's involvement in sexual affairs increased, his personality changed, becoming erratic and unpredictable. There were many signs; yet I ignored, even excused, the many symptoms that were screaming out to me that something was dreadfully wrong. In a sense, I betrayed my best self, the self that truly wanted and deserved happiness, by finding excuses for the many changes in Ted's personality instead of searching for their true meaning.

One of the most significant changes I noticed in Ted was his extreme fatigue. In the first years of our marriage he was a highly energetic person, alive with many interests. He was always active—fixing things around the house, working in the garden, rarely still a moment. Suddenly he was always tired.

During this time his behavior changed even at social events. When we attended a gathering of our friends or even a company party, Ted would end up asleep, stretched out on a sofa or collapsed on the floor. The behavior became a joke among our associates.

"Let's see where Ted will fall asleep tonight!" I laughed, and excused his somnolence, because I had become a typical co-dependent who explained away his behavior. "His job is so demanding," I explained, "He leaves for work at 5:30 every morning and doesn't get home until 6:00 in the evening, and he very frequently has evening meetings. The pressures are tremendous."

On one level I believed what I was saying. One reason Ted slept so much was that he was genuinely tired, but for reasons far different than I explained to myself and our friends and associates. Deception, like any kind of stress, uses a great deal of energy, and now I realize Ted was exhausted from the effort of always "covering his tracks," and of suppressing the shame he must have felt about his activities. I was correct when I said he was tired because of the pressures on him, but the pressures were not coming from his corporate colleagues. He confided to me years later, that he knew that he used sleep as an escape mechanism. If he were asleep, he wouldn't have to deal with me, our relationship, our children or problems of any kind. As his personal life became more and more chaotic, sleep was a way to avoid reality.

Addicts of all kinds are people who feel a great need to escape from the circumstances of their lives. Often they cannot face past events of their lives, including relationships with parents and hurtful childhood experiences that caused excessive fear and frustration. Addicts are also people who find difficulty dealing with any negative experience in adult life, from a rude salesclerk to a boss who is overly demanding. Addicts usually don't want to admit or experience their own negative feelings of anger, fear, guilt and frustration, however, so they seek escape from all the negative circumstances and emotions of their lives. One of their escapes is the object of their addiction—gambling, alcohol, sex, drugs, even shopping. By indulging in the addiction, the addict totally, but temporarily, can erase all perceived stress in his or her life.

Although I never let myself recognize that Ted's excessive sleep was avoidance, I did recognize avoidance in another big change in Ted—sudden lack of eye contact. I had been attracted to Ted in the first place partly because of his electric green eyes. I liked that he made so much eye contact and that his eyes were so full of expression and meaning.

But suddenly Ted stopped making eye contact; the expression was no longer there, not for me or for others close to him. The change did not go unnoticed. "You have darting eyes," others commented, and more than one friend implied that shame could be a reason for restless eyes.

As studies on alcoholism and other addictions repeatedly point out, shame, low self-esteem, and anxiety are the shared experiences of every addict. No one is proud of engaging in excessive, compulsive behavior, whether drinking or sexual involvement. Coping with the shame of his or her behavior becomes a demanding necessity for any addict.

I didn't recognize the shame, but I was very aware of Ted's lack of eye contact. In my personal and professional life I regard eye contact as very important to communication, and I felt annoyed when Ted no longer made eye contact with me. His eyes spoke loudly to me, "I don't want to deal with you. I'm not interested. I don't want to work on our relationship."

On the occasions when he did look at me, what I saw was an icy cold glare behind which was only vacancy. Then I would be the one to refuse to make eye contact. Although I did not acknowledge either Ted's apparent hatred or avoidance, I betrayed myself by not openly confronting him about the changes I saw in his eyes.

In my denial I avoided another explanation for his darting eyes. In the jargon of sexual addiction, Ted was constantly "cruising" with his eyes, looking for his next sexual conquest. I can picture him standing in the social hall of our church, his eyes darting around the room with an expression that was almost haunted. When I was curious enough to look in the direction he stared I invariably saw a woman. Even then I sensed he was fantasizing, but I didn't know he was plotting. Only much later did I understand that even at church Ted was constantly searching for new sexual partners.

Cruising is one of the ultimate activities for the desperate sex addict because he or she must have a constant supply of sexual partners at all times. The best-known locale for cruising is a singles' bar, but the true sex addict is *constantly* cruising at parties large and small, at church, on the job, even at home with guests. At the time I was oblivious to Ted's cruising, but I can now look back and see it quite clearly.

In crowds, Ted inevitably gravitated toward women. At any kind of social gathering he would "zero in on" an attractive woman and engage her in animated conversation. Many times he would sit with a woman at a party, laughing and relaxed while intently involved in discussion. He would certainly make eye contact in these situations, looking deeply into the woman's eyes and often touching her shoulders. At times these encounters developed into back rubs. Never would he have that sort of intense discussion with a man. I did ask myself why he always chose a woman for conversation, but betrayed myself again by not trying to answer my own question. For the most part, I saw what was happening, and I chose to ignore it.

Cruising involves subtle body language and verbal innuendo: a slight touch that lingers a bit too long, a sideways glance with a wry smile, a slightly off-color joke in combination with a touch or a glance or a smile.

Later, Ted revealed that whenever he met an interesting new woman he would automatically position himself to be in her line of vision, sometimes touching her as though by accident. He often made suggestive remarks to see how she would react. "I could always tell when a woman was interested," he said. He admitted that he particularly employed these strategies with a new substitute secretary at work, sending out as many messages as possible, fishing for a response. Our friends acknowledged having noticed such signals in our social life, but at the time I simply ignored the uneasy feeling I had when Ted's behavior seemed inappropriate.

Another change I noticed was Ted's increasing preoccupation and obliviousness to what was going on around him. He would sit for hours staring into space, seemingly less and less able to tune in to conversations meant to include him.

An incident during a visit to our hometown one summer was striking. I was talking with my mother about my family and she told me something funny about my Aunt Camilla.

"Isn't that just like Camilla?" I laughed, but he looked blank.

"Camilla who?" he asked. I was astounded. Ted had known my Aunt Camilla and her idiosyncrasies for years and we had laughed together about her adventures many times. It annoyed me that he wasn't interested enough to give our conversation his attention, but I stifled my irritation and once again said nothing.

Ted's lack of attention was more and more apparent at our family dinner table. "What?" he would respond blankly when one of our daughters said something to him.

"Oh, never mind," she would reply.

"What is the matter with him that he can't pay attention to his family?" I would ask myself, for he seemed incapable of tuning in to the needs and interests of the girls. Yet I never confronted him during this time, never asked him why he wasn't listening.

Ted's obliviousness to conversation extended beyond our family to our friendships. For many years we had theater tickets with friends and after seeing a play we enjoyed analyzing the performance and critiquing the production. Ted had been a lively participant in the discussions, expressing his opinions with vitality and wit. Gradually however, he withdrew until he would sit, morose and silent, while the other couple and I carried on our discussion. After attending a production of *A Midsummer Night's Dream*, I recall being particularly thrilled by the lavish costumes and brilliant color of the production. Ted reacted as though I were exclaiming about the merits of a new floor wax. His silence made me angry.

"Ted is becoming a dull and uninteresting person," I told myself bitterly. Yet I never questioned *why* he was becoming so detached.

When I began to study addictive behavior, I learned that a sexual addict becomes progressively more fearful of and isolated from normal contact with family and friends. This isolation is consistent with the withdrawal characteristic of any kind of addictive behavior. As the addict becomes more and more involved with any addiction, relationships with family and friends become less feasible and less important. Frequently the addict becomes totally obsessed with his or her addiction, to the exclusion of personal relationships altogether. The movie, *"Days of Wine and Roses,"* often hailed by professionals as a realistic portrait of alcoholism, depicts this obsession at the end of the film. When Lee Remick's character is presented with a clear choice between her family and the bottle, she chooses the bottle, as the flashing of the neon sign outside her seedy hotel room emphasizes the harsh isolation imposed by her choice.

Sexual addiction is different from other addictions because bodily contact with other people is a part of the addiction; yet the true sex addict does not form deep, lasting relationships with his sex partners. The obsession is with sex itself — with the conquest, the adventure, the defiance of society's rules — and never with a particular partner for any extended period of time. In spite of his or her numerous affairs, the sex addict is as isolated as the hard drug addict is a slave to his needle.

In addition to obsession with the addiction, another motivation for the addict's isolation is guilt. At some level he or she recognizes that the behavior is unacceptable, that he or she is disappointing others and not living up to their expectations. Rather than deal with this disappointment and the guilt it entails, the addict finds it easier to avoid personal relationships as much as possible.

Ted also became oblivious to me and to my appearance. He no longer noticed what I was wearing or how my hair was styled. He failed to compliment me on my appearance, even when I thought I looked my best. I "had my colors done," and I delighted in sewing outfits for myself with my personalized palette, but Ted was blind to my efforts. He heard others compliment me in his presence, but never said a word himself.

"I'm not very important to him," I told myself, "He doesn't care about me very much anymore." I never confronted him, however, choosing once again to ignore the fact that our relationship was deteriorating.

As Ted's illness progressed, he had waning interest in all the activities we had shared in the beginning of our marriage. He became more and more reluctant to work around the house, and began to complain about routine tasks, such as mowing the lawn. He began to argue with me in strange, erratic ways regarding the maintenance of our property.

We had a diseased fir tree in one corner of the lawn. Ted agreed with me that the tree should be examined, but the day the nurseryman was scheduled to come, Ted became very angry and canceled the appointment. "I'll take care of the tree by spraying and pruning it," he said. But he didn't do anything to take care of the tree and eventually it died. The Ted of our earlier years would have done everything possible to keep that tree from dying.

Another dramatic change in our relationship was the disappearance of playfulness. Early in our marriage we played like kittens, and we both loved competitive games of all kinds. Although Ted usually won at ping pong, I could beat him occasionally. Then he would tease me and chase me, threatening revenge. We enjoyed the same sort of friendly competition at other games, but gradually the raucous fun was draining from our marriage. I decided we were simply growing older. Lives filled with responsibility and duties sapped our energy. Both of us had loved to play with the girls. However, when I became playful and tussled with them, Ted would stand back with stern annoyance. "This is no good," he would say, "Someone is going to get hurt." He would then play with them in the same roughhousing manner, but he would get too rough. Sometimes someone did get hurt, such as the time our youngest received some serious rug burns on her elbows as a result of his roughness.

Losing humor and the ability to be playful is a particularly telling sign of personality trouble. When a person becomes unable to laugh at himself and his problems, he loses an important coping mechanism and may find himself overwhelmed by the seriousness of life. The childlike qualities of wonder, joy and spontaneity are frequently the qualities that give meaning to life. Without them life can seem increasingly dismal. Although I didn't fully understand the significance of Ted's growing lack of playfulness, when I noticed it I sensed that this loss was an indication of trouble. True to my pattern of not wishing to disrupt our family, however, I kept this sense of foreboding a secret.

I knew that Ted and I no longer shared as much as we once had, but I continually found an explanation for the fact that we were growing apart. "He's afraid of intimacy," I convinced myself. "He had no role models for it, and he doesn't know how to be intimate." It was my observation that Ted's family had lacked strong bonds of sharing and understanding. His parents had not enjoyed a close relationship, nor was Ted ever close to his brother, his only sibling. I used my knowledge of his family's lack of intimacy as an excuse for his withdrawal, not admitting that it was an insufficient explanation for a *change* in his behavior. I chose not to remember that we once had shared a very close, intimate relationship.

At the same time I convinced myself that Ted was afraid of intimacy, I accepted his developing close friendships with many other women. He referred to these women as *"true friends."* They were people with whom he could discuss personal problems and I was happy for him that he had these friendships. He had no close male friends, however. Somehow

I did not recognize the connection between the breech in our marriage and these other female relationships. I knew how much my friendships meant to me, and some of my friends were men. "Ted needs friends too," I rationalized. What did it matter if they were male or female?

It now amazes me that I failed to recognize the contradiction in my thinking about Ted's personality changes and behavior. Yet co-dependents of addicts typically juggle many such contradictions. Intensely eager to make the relationship work, the spouse of an addict will rationalize behavior in a hundred different ways, never perceiving a single discrepancy among any of the rationalizations. A co-dependent will thus add his or her own deceptions to those presented by the addict; the vision of reality becomes more clouded than ever, the secrets ever more deeply buried.

One of Ted's *"true friends"* was the woman with whom he had his first affair, Eleanor Butterfield. After he told me he had ended the sexual relationship, he explained he wanted to continue a friendship with this woman because they shared a great deal professionally, particularly an interest in telecommunications trends. I was convinced the relationship was no longer physical, but strictly professional. Much later I learned that Ted and this woman were lovers off and on for years.

Another of his *"true friends"* was an occasional visitor to his office from another floor. He recounted to me the problems of her second divorce and the difficulties she was having with her sons. "If I were single," he said, "I'd never date a woman who had children." Later I found out that Ted and the woman were lovers for five years.

What did he mean by his strange remarks to me — that he would never think of marrying this woman if our marriage should end? Or did he mean that if he were single and interested in finding another relationship, he wouldn't waste his time with this woman and have to deal with her concerns about her children? I told myself at the time that I was pleased he seemed to listen so empathetically to her problems, even though I *must* have thought the comments were strange.

To my knowledge, none of Ted's *"true friends"* is still important in his life. Characteristically, the sex addict is incapable of sustaining close relationships. He or she will present the *appearance* of intimacy, of understanding and caring, but these emotions will be short-lived. Following the excitement of conquest and the sexual fix, the focus of the sex addict turns to a new object.

During the time I hid these secrets from myself, Ted talked a great deal about women in a general way, often to no particular purpose that I could discern. One day as I was in the laundry room he passed by me after putting the lawn mower away. "You know," he said, "I don't know why a single woman would want to stay in a house."

"Where did that remark come from?" I thought to myself, but wouldn't let myself answer the question. Later I wondered if Ted had made some household repairs for his lover, after they had been to bed together at her house. No doubt his remarks to me were hints or clues as to his relationships, but I steadfastly ignored the connections.

There were more blatant clues to Ted's sexual relationships. One was an incident at the airport, the same place I received intimations of his first affair many years before. Once again, Ted returned from a business trip; once again, I met him as the airport. This time however, he was not expecting me. I decided on the spur of the moment to go and meet him, bringing our five-year-old daughter with me. We played a game as the gate disgorged its passengers: who will be the first to see Daddy? Neither of us was the winner because the stream of passengers stopped and Ted had not emerged. I was puzzled. Surely I had the correct arrival information. We waited as I considered possible scenarios. Had he missed his flight? Had he been taken ill aboard the plane?

Suddenly, Ted appeared at the gate, talking and laughing with a red-haired woman in a tan overcoat whom I had never seen before. His eyes met mine and then our daughter's, but they showed not a flicker of recognition. Instead, he walked on with the other woman, continuing his animated conversation. I fell into step beside him, our five-year-old trotting along after me, holding my hand. Ted ignored us as we headed down the concourse. Finally, the woman turned to me, obviously realizing who I was.

"Oh, I just enjoy Ted so much!" she said. After retrieving her baggage, she left us at the baggage claim and headed for her parked car. The three of us rode home in almost complete silence.

Now I wanted to confront Ted. Was I at last beginning to reveal the secret to myself? "There was some reason you two were the last ones off the plane last night," I finally made myself say to Ted the next day. He didn't answer me, and I said no more then. Perhaps I had expected a confession, but when it wasn't forthcoming I was stymied. Again I dropped the matter, and pushed the secret back into the recesses of my mind. Perhaps I was becoming too weary to confront him again.

A few weeks later we were invited to the home of Melanie Stern. I recognized the name Ted had mentioned before — the very woman who had been with Ted at the airport. I was not pleased at the dinner invitation and didn't want to be reminded of her existence. Ted was obviously looking forward to the evening with pleasure, but his remarks about the prospective social engagement were strange.

"Her husband is very seductive," he told me, "You will probably really fall for him."

"Do you know him well?" I asked.

"I've never met him, but she told me all about him. Apparently, every woman who meets him falls in love with him."

I did not let myself even consider the implications of her intimate revelation, once again keeping secrets from myself.

It was an unpleasant evening. Contrary to Ted's prediction, I did not find my host attractive, nor my hostess charming. She was giddy and giggly. Conversation was shallow and forced. I was delighted when the evening was over; the invitation was never repeated nor reciprocated.

I now believe that Ted was pushing me toward the husband with his suggestion that I would "fall for him." As I later studied sexual addiction, I learned that a sex addict will often try to encourage his or her spouse into extramarital sexual activities of one kind or another. If the addict is successful in fostering this behavior, he can condone and continue his own behavior and the sexual addiction is validated, relieving some of the addict's sense of shame. Other types of addicts will exhibit similar behavior, attempting to promote the same activity in the spouse. As misery loves company, so the addict loves to share his or her addiction. At the time however, I still did not suspect that this was Ted's motive in commenting on his lover's appealing spouse. I wouldn't even let myself consider that he was having an affair with the wife.

Another obvious clue I refused to let myself recognize was a gift from one of Ted's lovers. It was a tape of folk/rock music, and I discovered it in Ted's car. Such music had always bored Ted. He loved classical music and almost never listened to music of any other kind.

When I found the tape I asked him where it came from. He told me that it was a gift from a woman he had recently seen frequently. She was helping him rewrite his resume and she thought he might enjoy the tape. When I listened to the tape I found the songs quite sexually suggestive. Still I refused to let myself wonder why she would give him a tape with such songs on it.

After I learned the truth about Ted's behavior, I realized a huge inconsistency in it. He had been exploiting the woman who gave him the music tape. He was exhibiting a romantic interest in her while wanting to receive her help in advancing his career. On the other hand, when Mary Berg, another one of Ted's lovers sought his professional help, he felt used. Instead of helping her, he became angry and felt exploited.

"She just wants to *use* me," he said.

Exploitive behavior, as well as inconsistent behavior, is common among addicts of all kinds. Addicts habitually "use" people because they have an unhealthy sense of give and take and of appropriateness in relationships.

Lack of trust in relationships also can be one of the factors that drives an addict to his addiction in the first place, and relationships become less healthy once the addiction has become established.

Music was involved in another incident, an invitation to our thirtieth high school reunion. By the time we received the invitation I was quite sure I didn't want to attend.

"Go ahead and go if you want to," I told Ted when he asked me about the event. He did attend and returned to our home to tape some Fifties music. He explained that he was sending the tape to a mutual friend of ours, Charlotte Manning, whom he had seen at the reunion. Ted had spent quite a bit of time with her at the event, even riding around all night in her car with her after the reunion party.

Once again I could not come to terms with the truth about the nature of the relationship. After so many signs, hints and clues, I believe my self-esteem had eroded to the point that I might not have questioned Ted had he led a woman into our house and up the stairs to our bedroom.

Part of me seemed to conspire with Ted to keep secret the explanation of his strange behavior. In the face of strident evidence of Ted's woman-chasing, I played ostrich, hiding myself from the reality. I refused to acknowledge the life-altering secret I most dreaded, which for me still had no name that Ted might have a sex addiction. But my behavior only intensified the problem. I knew I deserved a good relationship and a fulfilling home life, but these satisfactions eluded me. I felt unspoken shame for having chosen this person for my mate. Only much later would I recognize that I was not responsible for his illness.

I understand why I couldn't face my situation, especially now that I have counseled co-dependents who have behaved exactly as I did. For Ted and me, denial was a means of survival. A co-dependent of any type of addict is living in a surreal, chaotic world which makes no sense and which is overwhelmingly destructive. The co-dependent dimly perceives that the entire structure of life must change, if the behavior he or she senses is true. Either the addict must reform or life for the co-dependent must be re-structured without the addict. Realizing either alternative is fraught with pain, with fear of change and of being alone. Thus the co-dependent takes refuge in the protection of denial, refusing to admit what, at some level, he or she knows to be true. My denial trapped me in a maze of secrets, lies and deceptions. It paralyzed me.

Chapter IV Exercise

Has this chapter given you new insight about betrayal? Do you think there have been times that you have looked the other way? Take some time to finish these sentences:

I remember one time when:

_____
_____
_____
_____
_____
_____
_____
_____
_____
_____

I just can't believe that :

_____
_____
_____
_____
_____
_____
_____
_____
_____
_____

Notes

Chapter V

Family Secrets

"Your goal is to find out who you are." - *Course in Miracles*

"Mom, stop lying about dad's behavior. I've known for a long time that he's been having affairs." Her words were shocking but to the point. She had never said them while living at home, but now she was asking to return home. This daughter, now living in Albany, had married very young and now had two children. Her marriage was falling apart and she needed to leave it, but had no resources to live on her own. She had phoned to ask if she could come home.

"Yes, you can come home," I responded, "but you have to know that your father and I are having a very difficult time right now."

It was at that point she divulged the suspicions and knowledge she'd had about her father. For years she had silently questioned why her father was gone so much, particularly to so many night meetings. What a burden this child had carried for so long! She had believed that if she had revealed the secret, it could have caused the family to break up.

It became her secret to bear in her early adolescence when I was out of town attending a meeting. Ted asked her and her sisters to collude in his secret activities. During adolescence, a very vulnerable time in their lives, our daughters learned the truth about their father's sexual behavior: their father was cheating on their mother.

Ted told the girls, Caroline, Lorraine, Rebecca and Amanda, ages sixteen, fourteen, nine and seven, that he felt they were old enough to stay alone while he went to our cabin for some quiet time by himself. They watched mystified as he packed food for the trip: two steaks, two potatoes, enough wine for a party. They also overheard him making arrangements over the phone to meet someone. Then they confronted him, telling him they were very uncomfortable that he was going to the cabin with someone else.

"Don't tell your mom. I'll tell her myself after she gets home."

Ted left for his rendezvous, but, as he told me years later, he never made it. The woman he was going to meet had an unexpected complication and couldn't come after all because the family she had arranged to keep her children were unable to do so. Ted then called the girls from her house and told them he was returning home because of car trouble.

Thus, Ted had asked the girls to deceive me, then deceived them about what really happened. Typical of an addict's behavior, his addiction took precedence over family responsibility. This incident contained the pattern of secrets within secrets and lies within lies, which came to characterize our family life. Because, as I was keeping secrets from myself, the entire family was being brought into the pattern.

To our daughters, the discovery of their father's infidelity was as if he had fired a shotgun while aiming at one person in a crowd. The target is likely to be wounded, but stray shot will injure others in the group. Our two eldest daughters suffered injuries affecting their own lives for years to come. Both of them chose partners to date and marry who were very much like their father. Both divorced after short marriages.

Children faced with a parent's infidelity fear the breakup of the family. If they acknowledge the secret, they are afraid it will cause the parents to divorce. Even though neither the infidelity nor the divorce is their fault, children carry guilt that they were somehow responsible. Thus, the trauma of parental infidelity presents an overwhelming amount of insecurity and anxiety for the children. The problem is accentuated for adolescents when their own sexuality is super-charged and confusing. It can be very frightening to observe their parents' inability to maintain sexual control as they are just learning about and investigating their own sexuality.

Children and adolescents are alert to whatever is going on between the parents. They are barometers of a family's health. Hoping to keep the family unit intact, children will act out to try to turn the parents' focus back to them, thus distracting the parents from each other.

Although they might not have been able to express their knowledge, our two oldest daughters knew about the tension between Ted and me. Pushing our family limits by returning home late, cutting classes at school and ignoring our concern for keeping good grades, they diverted my attention to the two of them and away from the problems in my relationship with Ted. These were important issues for me, and I thought for Ted, as well, but he didn't show as much concern. So their conduct kept a conflict simmering between us over how to be good parents of teenagers. For some time they succeeded in the goal of keeping the family unit intact. My concern about them did keep me from facing the problems that ultimately dissolved my marriage.

The girls were confronting an issue that almost always surfaces with infidelity: loyalty. Which side should they take? If they keep the secret, they are in collusion with the offending parent. If they tell, they put themselves in the role of caregivers for the wronged parent. Neither position is comfortable. In our daughters' case, because they were being used by their father to participate in the conspiracy, they chose not to confide in me until much later.

Secret-keeping between a parent and children regarding infidelity can have a marked effect on everyone's relationships. Although the girls did not tell me about the cabin incident until long afterward, Ted was always afraid they would. To placate them, he became more eager than ever to take *their* part in any argument they had with me. To keep me deceived about his behavior, he caused a rift in the relationship between me and my teenage daughters at a pivotal time in their lives. The rupture in our family was thus augmented by lies, deception and exploitation, and all of us kept our secrets.

Our daughters should have been allowed to negotiate the difficult tasks of adolescence, which include entering the second phase of separation from their parents. In order to negotiate this separation in a healthy, safe way, a stable family environment is important. The girls needed to have some assurance that their parents would be fine after they separated from them and left the home. Our family did not engender that kind of confidence.

The girls' acting out during this time created constant tension between Ted and me. Ted always sided with the girls. One source of disagreement in our family was what to do with my parents' special occasion gift money. The girls wanted to spend all the money, but I knew that my parents' intent was to help them learn money management, including saving for college or other long-term goals. Although I carefully explained this to the girls, Ted invariably took their side and all of them would oppose me. Finally, I would give in, annoyed that Ted interfered with my own parents' wishes and angry that I was made to play the "heavy" in these disagreements.

I was also the "bad guy" with regard to discipline. As they reached adolescence, I became quite concerned about the girls' appearance of promiscuous behavior. Our two older daughters matured physically at an early age. By the time each was in the sixth grade, she had a fully-developed figure. Naturally, this physical maturity attracted older boys. By the time each girl turned twelve, she was attracting boys of sixteen and seventeen. Soon the oldest was sneaking out of the house at night in order to meet with boys at the nearby McDonald's. Within a couple of years, the younger joined in to keep up with her older sister.

Ted saw no problem with the girls dating much older boys. I felt the girls should at least have guidance in these relationships, and I wanted to establish rules about how often they could see the boys and how late they could stay out. Ted always disagreed with me on setting reasonable limits. I felt strongly enough on the matter that I set rules for them myself, but enforcing them was impossible. Ted refused to support me, shifting the conflict from our relationship to our children.

The confrontations I had with the girls in those days were terrible. They expressed open hatred, using hurtful words and regarding me with disdainful looks. "Bitch" was one of the milder names they called me. Ted refused to support me, simply shrugging his shoulders when I appealed to him.

The girls' vicious attacks on me and Ted's indifference were just another secret in the dark, carefully locked closet of our family's life. Ted did not want me to discuss their behavior with my friends. In fact, he became angry if he found out that I talked to anyone about family matters, saying that our problems were strictly private and should never be discussed outside the family. Ted wanted to project a family image of perfection. In time, the girls also became angry if I talked to anyone about our family problems. Increasingly, I felt isolated. Because I was reluctant to share my distress with anyone outside the sources of the distress, I also became ambivalent, questioning and doubting myself. Was I at fault? Did I have the wrong "take" on my relationship with Ted and the girls? Was I overreacting? Was I too rigid?

This lack of communication with outsiders, even extended family, served to reinforce the unhealthy, closed system in our family. In *Peoplemaking*, Virginia Satir notes that one of the best ways to deliberately create a closed system is to limit interaction with the outside world. By keeping destructive behavior secret and refusing to allow it to be scrutinized by anyone, we intensified the destructive patterns in our family. Our power struggle was a secret we kept from nearly everyone who knew us.

The triangulation of the relationship between Ted and our two older daughters was their collusion, which kept me out. It was never more apparent than on one of our family trips to our wilderness cabin near Adirondack Park. They were young teenagers. The evening before we were to leave for the cabin Ted made a casual announcement. "The girls' boyfriends will be going with us tomorrow," he said.

I was incredulous. "You told the girls they could invite them without even consulting me?" I asked. Ted simply shrugged, and I realized I had been put on the outside once again. They had an agreement, and I hadn't known anything about it.

"Why didn't you ask me if it was OK?" I persisted, but again Ted didn't answer. "I'm not sure I have enough food, for one thing," I went on.

I *wasn't* sure about the food and I couldn't believe Ted's lack of consideration about the problem of two extra mouths to feed. Of course, the food wasn't the biggest issue. I was not comfortable with our daughters' relationships with their boyfriends and I wasn't happy about having them accompany us on a family weekend.

Ted must have known how I felt, and so postponed mentioning their inclusion until the last minute. The boys had already been invited and the girls were very excited about having them come along. If I refused to let them come at this point, I would be a bad guy of the first order, and I knew it.

I felt I had no choice but to pack whatever extra food I had and make the best of the situation. I had never felt so much a victim of a conspiracy.

After we reached the cabin, however, I began to feel even more alarmed. One of the boys began touching our daughter in ways I felt were most inappropriate. As soon as I could, I took Ted aside and told him of my concerns.

"Haven't you noticed?" I asked. "Haven't you seen the way he is touching her?" Ted gave me a chilling look that spoke volumes.

"How else will they learn?" he asked rhetorically. He said it with such authority that I was intimidated into silence. Perhaps I *was* hopelessly behind the times in my thinking about manners, morals and sexual activity among young people. Once again I felt alone and unsupported.

Much, much later I learned that my fears were well founded. Both older girls were sexually active early, and both escaped pregnancy as young teenagers only by incredible luck. Yet their sexual behavior, like their father's, was a well-kept secret from both me and the outside world.

Another incident involving the girls and their boyfriends clearly revealed the instability of most of the members of our family. We had taken a trip back to our hometown for a visit. While we were there our teenage daughters, thirteen and fifteen at the time, struck up a friendship with two much older boys who had rented a house and were living there alone. After we returned home, the girls made plans to run away from our home and return to our hometown to live with these boys.

I was working in our yard when suddenly I heard a thud against the front fence. I went around the house to investigate and saw a large suitcase leaning against the fence. I knew trouble was brewing and decided to keep it from erupting until Ted came home, perhaps hoping one more time that he would give me some much-needed support with the girls. I made myself prominent in the front yard, weeding flowerbeds that were already immaculate. When Ted pulled into the driveway, I met him before he got out of the car.

"Something is going on," I said and told him about the suitcase. Together we confronted the girls. They readily admitted their plans. They were to be picked up by an older friend with a driver's license who would take them to the bus station. There they could get tickets to our hometown. One daughter accompanied me to the bank earlier in the day to observe me as I made a withdrawal. She had returned to make a $1,000 withdrawal from her own account and because our family was well known in the community, no one at the bank questioned the transaction.

We aborted their plans immediately. I left to take the money back to the bank, leaving Ted with the girls. I assumed he would talk with them, try to help them see the foolishness of their plans. Instead he staged a dramatic and horrifying scene. He made the girls go with him to the garage, took down one of his hunting guns and pointed the gun at his head.

"If you try to leave, I will shoot myself," he told the girls. "You can't leave me or I'll die," Ted said to the girls.

Rather than facing whatever circumstances had made them want to leave home, he used a monstrous threat to keep them there and on his side. Thus, he forced them into the role of caregivers when they needed to be attending to their own adolescent tasks.

One of them told me that she still has a vivid and terrible picture of her father standing in the garage threatening to shoot himself. As for me, I had no idea the girls were carrying this secret until after their father and I were divorced.

I now wish I had summoned the strength to insist we all go for family counseling at that point. But I was weary and wary. Had I known about Ted's paralyzing suicide threat in front of the girls, I'm certain I would have insisted. Though I had managed to persuade Ted to go for counseling a couple of times before, we had never made any progress. Whenever it was suggested that Ted could change some behaviors, he immediately quit.

A snarl of secrets such as we endured is endemic to the family life of any unhealthy or dysfunctional family, but it is particularly tangled in the family of the sexual addict.

The addict usually needs to leave the house in order to pursue his addiction. Leaving requires lies and these lies soon proliferate.

Just as Ted wanted to keep secret the problems we were having with the girls, he also wanted to hide the fact that our marriage bond had weakened. From the time of his first affair, the trust between us began to erode. This erosion of trust and commitment was reflected in our sex life that became less and less satisfying. My ardor grew cold. During our lovemaking, I experienced intrusive thoughts about the woman with whom he'd had the affair. As I look back, I realize the fun and playfulness was disappearing from our sex life, which was becoming mechanical and forced. No longer did loving remarks punctuate our interaction. A coldness set in, and I suspect that Ted's mind was always somewhere else when we were making love. During sex, fantasizing is quite normal and healthy; however, the complete lack of any emotional connection between us during sex was *not* either healthy or normal. The growing rift between us, seen most clearly in our joyless sex life, was a secret that Ted would never have wanted the outside world to suspect.

During one memorable trip to our cabin, the tension between us reached crisis proportions. He made sexual advances to me as soon as we arrived at the cabin, but I was in no mood for sex. I wanted to sit on the couch and talk while he held me. I wanted to try to understand the reasons for his behavior and to recapture the rapport we had once shared.

"I have no feelings for you," he said abruptly.

"Then...why do you want sex?" I asked.

He got up suddenly and stomped out of the room. He was gone for three or four hours. When he returned he was visibly agitated and upset. Again he started making sexual advances and I was puzzled.

"What are you feeling now? What do you feel for me?" I asked.

"Goddamn it, woman, can't you understand that sex is how I *show* feeling?" he shouted, as he jumped up and ran outside.

I followed him to the top of a cliff near our cabin. He stood close to the edge, threatening to jump and waving good-bye. Then he fell on the rocks at the top of the cliff, screaming. I went over to him and touched him gently on the shoulder and he calmed down.

As I was seeing a therapist at the time, I related this incident to him. "Don't you see?" my therapist asked. "He has to hurt you before he can have sex with you. Love and sharing are not part of the agenda before sex." As he spoke, I realized that sex *had* become more and more hurtful. Sex had become a demand. It was a demand that not only changed our relationship, it demeaned me and sent me reeling into a further spiral of self-doubt and confusion.

"You *have* to satisfy me," Ted seemed to say with every sexual advance. If I wasn't in the mood, he pouted. "You don't care about me," was his attitude. "If you cared, you'd be sexually excited by me."

There was no longer any love in the act and Ted seemed close to rage when we had sex. It seemed to be a form of punishment for me and his anger made the act border on rape. I sensed the form that our sex together had taken, and I found it frightening.

One evening, as we were driving home, he began to make sexual advances toward me, along with negative comments about my many "inadequacies." As the car stopped at a traffic light, I opened the door and got out, refusing to let him continue to degrade me. I walked the few blocks to our house, arriving home shortly after he did. Neither of us mentioned the incident, but I had made the first move in twenty-eight years of marriage to stop his emotional and sexual abuse.

No one suspected the verbal, emotional and sexual abuse that had become such a part of our lives. Ted was still carefully maintaining his façade as a community builder, loving husband and father, and caring human being. If our small community on the outskirts of New York had a "Good Neighbor" award, Ted surely would have been nominated. He enjoyed doing helpful things for others. The snow blower always had a full tank of gas so he would be ready after each new snowfall to clear blocks of sidewalks. Being an early riser, he would have the walks cleared while many of the houses were still dark.

Cloaked with such a careful façade, no one could have known that our family life was in shambles or charged with deadly tension. Yet there were ways our family secrets were not nearly as secret as we all thought. Ten years after the death of my mother, her sister revealed to me that my mother had thought that Ted was having affairs. I wished that my mother had been able to confide her observation to me when she was alive. But I understand that she, too, had been protecting our relationship. In order to shield me, she kept her observation a secret from me. Although my mother's silence was with good intent, it was enabling, allowing the dysfunction to continue and helping to perpetuate both his affairs and my denial.

As painful and crazy-making as Ted's behavior was, a revelation from my oldest daughter brought a new round of despair. Five years after our divorce came the dreaded phone call — the one no mother ever wants to receive. One of my daughters called to ask if I would support her decision to undergo therapy to work on the possibility that she had been sexually abused. She was in her early 30's, the age many young women begin to experience memories of sexual abuse.

"Why do I wake up in the night in a fetal position on the very edge of my bed and have to get up and put on my clothes?" she asked, "Why do some noises startle me while others give me comfort?"

One more secret was revealed. Even after all I had been through I was incredulous about the revelation of incest in my own family. How could this have gone on under the roof of *our* home? Under my nose? I was devastated to learn this new horror about my husband's behavior, even though I knew by then that it was not uncommon among sex addicts.

New feelings of failure swelled within me: I was a mother who had not protected her child from sexual abuse. The feeling of hopelessness that this saga would never end sent me into renewed depression. Immediately I went into therapy in order to manage the rage and homicidal thoughts I was having. This time an antidepressant helped me through the despair.

"A mother's suffering can be as great as the child's who endured the abuse," said one professional to me. Now I knew that my husband not only betrayed his role as a husband but also his role as a father. He had misused his power as a parent by abusing his daughter. He taught her to sexualize relationships with men, and the insidious nature of the addiction had thus been passed on to the next generation. Thankfully, that was not the end of our daughter's story.

I was still in the Boston area in graduate school, so my daughter traveled to meet me. We took a road trip from Cambridge to New York to discuss her memories and concerns.

A large box of tissues was used up as we traveled. That collection of soggy tissues was the beginning of the healing of our relationship, the building of a strong bond between us. Thanks to her therapy and my studies, our eyes opened to the realities of sexual abuse. We were now able to focus on our relationship, to make sense of why she had raged at me for so many years, to understand her promiscuous behavior.

One of the symptoms of sexual abuse is rage toward the mother or other parent because that parent is not protecting the child from harm. The child believes that the parent who is not the abuser, usually the mother, knows what is happening and is doing nothing to protect the child and stop the incest. In some cases the mother does know, and does nothing out of fear or for some other reason. In my case, I did not know, at least not on a conscious level.

As for my daughter's promiscuous behavior, sexually abused children often begin to learn that sexual involvement is the way to gain attention and affection. A father may tell his child to keep the secret because they have this special relationship. Moreover, a father can convince a daughter that this is normal behavior.

By the time she went into therapy, my daughter was so ready to work on the issue that her time in therapy was very short. For example, when her therapist informed her that she would need to do intense raging at her mother, there was silence. "I have raged so long and hard at my mother she does not deserve any more of my wrath," she finally responded. Her anxiety and anger had dissipated.

Ultimately she shared with me one of her most insightful thoughts. "When you divorced dad, you gave me permission to divorce him also."

How beautiful our relationship is now; and how cheated I feel to have missed some very important years in both of our lives.

Later, in relating this to two close friends who are both mental health professionals, each confirmed their own observations regarding Ted's behavior. Wishing desperately to keep our family secrets, we all ultimately failed. By keeping the secrets we failed each other. As the dimension of the secrets grew, we failed even to keep the secrets. Although the cancerous secrets in our family life left us all with deep wounds, revealing the secrets led to solutions and, finally, to healing for my daughters and myself.

Chapter V Exercise

Have you forgotten what you appreciate or like about yourself? Have you been told that you are not good enough just the way you are and do you believe it? Take some time to cut pictures, words, phrases or symbols out of magazines that express what you appreciate about yourself. Glue them to a piece of posterboard and place it some where you can see it every day. This is a collage of the good things you are.

_____

_____

_____

_____

_____

_____

_____

_____

_____

_____

_____

_____

_____

_____

_____

_____

_____

Notes

_____

_____

_____

_____

_____

_____

_____

_____

_____

_____

_____

_____

_____

_____

_____

_____

_____

_____

_____

_____

_____

_____

_____

_____

Chapter VI

Sharing the Secrets with Others

"Never look down to test the ground before taking your next step; only he who keeps his eyes fixed on the far horizon will find the right road." — Dag Hammarskjold

"Surviving is important, but thriving is elegant."
Maya Angelou

Ted moved out in May of our 28th year of marriage. He told me that he had to leave to keep his sanity. To me, this meant he had decided that leaving me to live with another woman could solve his problem. The other woman had told him that her love could make him a different person. So Ted continued to believe that the solution was to be found outside himself, that happiness could be found in the outside world. He rejected any need for change within himself.

As soon as Ted left, I knew I had to be proactive. I contacted a number of friends who had been through divorces and asked for their opinions of the attorney they had used. After reviewing opinions on eight different attorneys, I chose three to interview in an attempt to find the best possible person to represent me. I decided that I would no longer be victimized; I would take control of my own life and choose my direction. This decision proved to have a powerful and positive effect on my journey toward healing.

All three attorneys I had chosen to interview were surprised when I arrived with a financial statement in hand. I had brought the statement because I was concerned about my financial future, and wished to see how each attorney would evaluate my prospects.

As I interviewed the three, I paid special attention to their behavior. One seemed apathetic, giving me the impression he would not defend a woman well. Another began typing papers while we were still meeting in the interview, making me feel she was rushing me. The attorney I chose listened and gave me advice. At the end of the interview hour, she asked if I were ready to serve divorce papers. She seemed to have empathy for the difficult days I had ahead of me, yet she also was able to stay on task and keep my financial wellbeing in focus.

Therapeutic as was my decision to hire an attorney, the two weeks of my search was a miserable time for me. I cried constantly, vacillating between tears of anguish and tears of rage. My body ached with tension, and I felt my blood pressure must be sky-high. I was unable to sleep more than an hour at a time, but I did not seek medical help.

I was afraid of my future as a single person, and very much afraid of what people would think of me, how they would react to me. I dreaded the thought of facing people and having to tell them what had happened to my marriage.

I spent much of the summer "facing dragons." The first thing I did was to return to Spencer, where Ted and I had grown up. There I visited close friends and relatives, both Ted's and mine. I told people the truth about my marriage and why it had ended. In contrast to my nightmares and fears that I would experience rejection and censure, everyone I visited was very supportive and nurturing. I stayed a week in our old hometown—talking, explaining and receiving support. There my healing began in earnest, as I felt revitalized by the strength and energy that I felt flowing from everyone I saw.

Next I traveled to see my favorite aunt, who had been like a second mother to me, especially after my own mother died. I told her my story, and she responded without judgment but with love, caring and the deepest empathy. I let myself be nurtured by her as we shared my secrets.

Close to home, the "dragons" were most fearsome. How would my friends react? Our all-church summer camp had been an annual event for our family for years, and Ted and I had both served on the planning committee. How would I feel attending as a single person? How would people react to my coming alone? I had shared my secrets with some of those who would be at camp, but others would not yet know what I was going through.

The camp "dragons" proved to be as benign as those I had faced earlier in the summer. I did not experience the same sort of fun I was used to having at camp, but I was resigned to the fact that this was not a carefree period of my life. I spent much of the time there with a very close friend — talking, talking, talking. We would go off to the meadow every afternoon; "going to the weeds," we called it. Others at camp were similarly understanding and nurturing. All these "dragons" were healthful and healing, soothing my wounds and calming my spirit.

Mine were the kind of false fears with which we human beings often torture ourselves. Imagining a bad experience is frequently far worse than the experience itself. "Cowards die many deaths, while brave men die but once," - Leo Rosten.

Releasing the fear by facing whatever is most dreaded can sometimes result in a surprisingly positive experience. Facing my "dragons" certainly taught me to be less afraid of what life had to offer.

I also feel especially fortunate about the support of my Presbyterian church. I later met other divorced people who experienced feelings of rejection or censure from church groups that had been a part of their lives when they were married. I did not share their experience in any way. I believe I am lucky to belong to a church that is accepting and which includes a large number of single people in its membership. My church is an ongoing source of support for me.

I continued to share the story of my secrets with those who had been my friends for years, but I did not stop there. I invited some people into my confidence who had been on the fringes of my life, such as acquaintances in my New Rochelle sisterhood. Some had gone through divorce themselves and brought the gift of empathy as I invited them in. Others brought gifts of care, support, encouragement and acceptance, as well as a revelation of how essential and beneficial it is to belong to a community.

However, as I returned to the home where Ted and I had lived together for twenty years, I suddenly felt very frightened about rebuilding my life alone. I was in middle age, with scar tissue not yet formed on many of the wounds of my dissolving marriage. I knew that I needed to find full-time employment to replace the part-time work I had enjoyed for so long. The thought of job hunting at my age was daunting. I began to look around for resources, and found a 10-week career development course.

The program focused on women in transition; women whose lives were changing because of divorce, widowhood, economic necessity, children growing out of the family, or other such circumstances. Some women turned to the courses simply because they *wanted* their lives to change. They felt a need for growth, but were uncertain about how to fulfill that need. This intensive course focused on finding emotional and practical tools for making a career change, or entering the job market for the first time. My class of twenty included a wide variety of women with diverse backgrounds. Ages ranged from mid-twenties to mid-sixties. Only four of us had completed college degrees. A few were divorced or widowed, but most were married and interested in changing the direction of their lives within their marriages. We were all seeking employment that would meet both our financial and our emotional needs.

Mornings were spent learning practical steps for career change. In these sessions we received assistance with resume writing and learned how we could translate skills acquired in volunteer work or in past job experience to other positions. We took a battery of personality and interest tests that helped us understand the kind of career and work environment in which we might be happiest.

In the afternoons we received emotional support for the changes we were trying to make in our lives. We encouraged one another while skillful leaders helped us discover the courage and other personality characteristics necessary to make the changes we were seeking. I left the program feeling, not that I had found all the answers, but that I was capable of finding the answers as time and experience presented them to me.

For me, it was the first step in healing my wounds by changing the direction of my life. I learned that I could take the skills I had acquired as a teacher and put them to use in another field, such as marketing or sales. I looked at fields I had never before considered, and found the idea of exploring new areas exciting.

Unfortunately, I later learned that the program no longer exists, but similar programs are available in many communities in places such as community colleges, university women's centers, YWCA's and other community organizations. If I were to find myself once again in the position of starting over, I would search for such a program.

Receiving job information and meeting other women trying to change their lives were valuable experiences, but perhaps the greatest need that this life-changing program filled for me was my need for a definite, practical agenda. It gave me a reason to get out of bed every morning, a place to go and information resources to help me travel the unfamiliar road on which I found myself.

Ultimately, my participation in this 10-week program was a start, but I needed more help than simply job counseling and support from other women in transition. My emotions were still in turmoil, and my predominant mood was depression. I still wasn't sleeping well at night, and I dragged myself through my days with little energy. I had trouble concentrating, felt that nothing in my life was worth doing, and doubted that I could again find joy in life. The idea of a new career was exciting, but I lacked the energy to pursue it. I knew enough about depression to recognize that I was experiencing it. I also knew that depression could be anger turned inward, and I wanted to find out if rage was at the root of my depression. I did not believe that I still blamed myself for Ted's behavior, but was I, deep inside, angry with myself? I wanted to explore my depression, discover how to deal with it and find out how I could get rid of it.

The logical person to turn to in my quest was a therapist; however, I hesitated to begin the search to find one. I had abandoned my own therapist when Ted and I had gone on our trip to Europe. My joint visits to Ted's therapist ended when he moved out. I was left without the support of a mental health professional. For some reason I didn't even ask my physician for help.

When I had stopped seeing my own psychiatrist in the city, a somewhat dour man in his sixties, I discovered that I was relieved not to have to go to him every week. I now feel that he had been part of the problem. He had seemed to me somewhat depressed himself, therefore giving me little sense that he could help me with *my* depression. He also pressed me to work on issues that I felt were only indirectly relevant. He pushed me to go back in my experience, returning to grieve over the deaths of my parents and little brother, but I felt I had sufficiently grieved for those terrible losses. I had even become involved in the work of a local hospice following the death of my father. My psychiatrist also indicated to me that he believed I had never had a good relationship with a man. He suggested I had chosen Ted because he was a man bound to let me down, as he believed other men in my life had. I disagreed with his assessment. I believed that my relationship with my father had been a good one and that I had several loving, caring uncles who also had provided me with good male relationships as a young girl. Furthermore, I enjoyed several good, platonic friendships with other men at the time. I respected my therapist, but I also respectfully disagreed with some of his diagnoses and suggestions.

Because of our differences and incompatibilities, my therapist and I seemed to pull in different directions the entire time I saw him. Any progress we made came very slowly. With him as my only experience, I might have rejected therapy altogether. However, my experience with the therapist Ted and I visited jointly had been quite the reverse.

Ted had chosen an excellent therapist, and I soon decided she was helping me more than Ted. Her attitude was cheerful and optimistic, giving me feelings of encouragement. Our visits made me feel that my life could change for the better. She helped me understand my feelings and interpret some significant dreams I was having during that period.

With help from this therapist, I had begun to understand that I was a creative, valuable person with a great deal to offer — someone who could survive and thrive by herself. I had begun to believe that I would be able to make important new decisions, and most importantly, that I was not to blame for Ted's problems and behaviors.

Yet, as much as I appreciated this therapist, however, I did not choose to return to her as I was beginning my new, single life. I wanted to start fresh with a new therapist unconnected with my past with Ted.

I did not search for a therapist in the same way I had made my search for a divorce attorney, with research, selection of several candidates and interviews. Like many people, I was unduly influenced by the mystique of the health professional. Too often, we approach shopping for a financial advisor or an attorney as we would shop for any business service, but do not apply the same standard to those who provide our health care. We mistakenly believe health care providers should be above the mundane scrutiny of shopping, expecting they all must be as competent as their commitment to care giving would suggest. I would wholeheartedly recommend shopping for a health care professional as diligently as one shops for anything else.

By sheer luck, I did manage to find an excellent therapist. She was a social worker, recommended by a friend. As a social worker, this therapist was trained in a different discipline than others I had consulted. My experience taught me that the discipline — psychiatry, psychology, social work or psychiatric nursing — is not nearly as important as personality, rapport and the manner in which the therapist helps the client address the issues.

I liked Ruth Starr immediately because of her empathy. By my third visit I was convinced she would be able to help me deal with my depression. I felt a wonderful rapport between us. She also forced me to look closely at all the possible causes for my depression and to sift through these factors one by one.

As my therapy slowly proceeded, I found other resources that also encouraged healing. One was a divorce support group, based on Bruce Fisher's book, *When Your Relationship Ends*. The weekly group meetings focused on Fisher's fifteen building blocks toward recovery from divorce. Although none of the other people in the group had faced the problem of sexual addiction in their marriages, I discovered that my feelings of depression and emotional unsteadiness were shared by almost everyone. It was marvelous to know that I *wasn't* going crazy. Many other people were on emotional roller coaster rides too!

From the tests we took every week, I learned that I was ahead of many participants in some areas. One of Fisher's first building blocks is self-esteem, and I found that I rated high in this area. I began to realize that I had been working hard to build my self-esteem ever since I learned of Ted's first affair. My work had paid off. I discovered I felt good about myself. The crippling guilt I had once felt about Ted's behavior had almost completely disappeared.

Another area where my rating was high was in my willingness to reach out and form new relationships. Although I definitely was not ready for a male-female romantic relationship, I was open to friendships with members of both sexes. Indeed, the acquaintance I began with two women in the divorce group blossomed into friendships that continued long after the group was over.

The testing also revealed to me areas I needed to work on, such as ridding myself of anger and disengaging from Ted. Even at the end of the support group course, I found that I carried a great deal of anger at Ted for all the hurt he had caused me. I was not only angry with Ted, but also angry with myself for tolerating his behavior all those years. As I became more aware of my anger, I could look at the reasons for my depression.

Anger was one of the main focal points in my therapy with Ruth. She helped me discover that I needed to love myself even when I was angriest, and that it was okay to feel anger. Conversely, all my life I had been taught that anger, especially rage, was unacceptable. I was aware that "pop" psychology viewed anger as acceptable, even healthy, but I still found it distasteful. Ruth helped me accept anger as a valid emotion. She taught me that perhaps the worst thing one can do with anger is to deny that it exists. The best thing to do is recognize it fully, then channel it properly.

Ruth helped me see that anger becomes destructive only when it is expressed inappropriately. Sometimes inappropriate expression of anger includes confronting the person who is the focus of your anger. For me, it was not appropriate to confront Ted. By now I had realized that he was probably incapable of controlling his sexual obsession. By the same reasoning, it was not appropriate for me to confront myself concerning my years of denial about Ted's behavior. I was powerless to change the way I had behaved in the past. Using my anger to berate myself was very destructive and an important component of my depression.

Ruth introduced me to the idea of using my anger creatively. She taught me that anger is energy and that I could use this energy for creative accomplishment. "How have you used your anger?" she would ask me at every session. As the weeks went by, I became proud of the answer I could give to her question. I began with simple accomplishments such as cleaning closets, using my anger literally to re-order my life.

Gradually, my projects became more ambitious. "I am painting my house," I told Ruth one day. I meant the outside of my house, which was a two-story home. I was very proud when I single-handedly completed this extensive project. I had used my anger to find the energy for the ambitious task.

"I cut down three large trees that were dead or diseased," I told Ruth another time. Among these trees was the fir tree that Ted had promised he would save. I succeeded in "playing lumberjack" without power tools, and once again, was proud of my accomplishment. I later planted new trees to replace the ones I had removed, and felt a surge of new life in me as well.

As I used my anger for these accomplishments, I realized that I was achieving other purposes. I was reclaiming the house and making it my own. I was disengaging from Ted by not having to depend on him to do the difficult physical work. I was seeing my ability to control my own life, and my self-confidence surged.

As I experienced new power in myself, I found another community resource that helped me confirm the strengths in my personality. This resource was a class in genology. It was not "genealogy," the study of my ancestors, but "genology," the study of the *personalities* of my ancestors. The idea was to find the vitality in my family tree, to focus on these inherent positive traits and see how I could incorporate them into my own life.

While I had some information about my forebears, a bit of research revealed more. I learned that my mother's side of the family included strong female "dynamos" who were excellent managers and organizers. My mother's grandfather had walked away from his family, leaving my great-grandmother to cope with raising her family alone. She succeeded in this difficult venture, aligning herself with other dynamic women in the family. On my father's side of the family, my grandfather returned to the United States nine times before he was able to settle permanently. His persistence paid off. He eventually became a respected member of his community with a family of nine children. His side of the family included several creative artists — writers, painters and musicians.

I also learned that my mother's side of the family included relatives in France and England who suffered from depression and alcohol problems, but because of the focus of the genology class I learned not to be dismayed by this information. I learned I could choose not to follow in the steps of ancestors who had such problems, but choose to adopt the strengths and accomplishments of my more successful forebears. I saw in my own life evidence of the vigor of my ancestors and the accompanying resilience that contributed to my healing.

Using the energy of my anger and finding my strengths were empowering, but I discovered that my depression was composed of more than anger alone. It included disappointment, frustration, grief and fear. Even if the anger were successfully addressed, the other destructive emotions would remain. Once again, Ruth assured me that my depression would not last forever, and she urged me to explore the depression by asking myself why I was feeling it. She encouraged me to give myself permission to *feel* my negative emotions as deeply as possible. One of my most productive days in therapy was the day she told me to go home and cry as long as I possibly could. I followed her direction and sobbed for hours. At the end of crying, I felt cleansed.

Ruth and I both knew that tears alone would not heal me, but recovery *was* taking place—slowly, gradually, often without my notice.

Community resources such as my 10-week course, my dreams, my work with my therapist, the support of friends and acquaintances, and the passage of time all helped me deal with the various components of my depression and the fears I had about sharing my secrets and giving up my marriage. The more I used my anger to strengthen myself, the better I felt about myself. The better I felt about myself, the more the anger dissipated. Disappointment, frustration, sorrow, and fear also were decreasing, but it was necessary to explore each emotion in detail to promote my healing.

Along the way I realized that my negative emotions were intimately connected to my reasons for staying in a marriage which I knew was not giving me what I wanted. I stayed because I could not accept the reality and face the fact that the man I married was someone I couldn't trust—that he no longer shared values that I still prized highly. When I finally opened my eyes to the reality of Ted's secrets, refusing at last to be blind to his behavior, my disappointment and frustration were inevitable. All my life I had cherished the idea of a good marriage, believing for a long time that I had one. To admit to the possibility that perhaps I had *never* had one was to be disappointed and frustrated. Gradually I began to realize that happiness and fulfillment are possible without marriage. I was a perfectly acceptable human being as a single person.

Confronting sorrow was also an inevitable part of letting go of my life as it had been, and my resulting grief was composed of many aspects. First, I grieved over the loss of the man I had married; the man I could trust, the man who had shared my values, the man I wanted him to be, or the man I thought he was. I also grieved that I was no longer a married person, the kind of person who had symbolized successful adulthood when I was growing up. I grieved the loss of my life with Ted, along with the loss of a future of our shared experiences. Each of these aspects of grief was composed of many layers. It was a long time before I peeled them all away.

One of my overwhelming fears about ending my marriage was my concern that my life with Ted and our mutual history would somehow be invalidated. Ruth helped me realize that the history of my life with Ted was still quite valid. I did not have to continue to share my life with him in order to appreciate the good times and the meaningful challenges and struggles we had shared in the past. These experiences would also be part of my life, and they would always be significant.

Another fear I had about leaving my marriage revolved around my dread of rejection and failure. Facing my dragons and discovering that they actually were friendly, not threatening, helped a great deal to dispel those fears. Yet I still felt a sense of failure that my marriage had ended. Very slowly I let go of this sense of failure, realizing that I had done everything I could to make the marriage work.

"Your life will never be the same," Ruth told me, "Because of these experiences, you will live the rest of your life differently. You are a changed person because of what has happened, but you can pick up the pieces and make a better life than you had before." I embraced Ruth's words, knowing on some level that they were true. I also knew that making a better life was a big job I had ahead of me.

My greatest fear of all focused on the future. In the aftermath of the divorce I was quite uncertain about my financial situation. I knew that I needed a full-time job, for emotional as well as financial reasons. I was not sure whether my interim financial resources would be sufficient while I pursued a new career that would be right for me. At the time, local economies were in a period of recession and jobs were scarce. The making of my new life began with a sense of panic. I was impatient with the tortoise pace of my job hunt.

"Can't you relax and just enjoy *being*?" Ruth asked. Relaxation *was* difficult. I was anxious to move on, to get past all the negative emotions and into a realm of positive accomplishment. Now I realize that Ruth was right. I was fortunate not to be able to move too quickly. Healing took time, and I needed to take that time to work on my emotional turmoil. I needed time for my anger, disappointment, frustration, grief and fear to be replaced by soothing and restoring experiences.

When my new job came, my recovery was not yet complete, and new work itself came with more frustrations. But at long last I was ready to move on.

Chapter VI Exercise

"Anger is a physical experience, a rush of energy and adrenalin meant to motivate, protect and empower for action." - Kathleen Fischer

Do you have anger that could give you energy and motivate you to take new directions in your life?

Take a piece of posterboard and write, New Directions at the top. Once again, go to the magazines and find pictures, words, symbols and phrases that represent new directions you would like to take in your life.

_____

_____

_____

_____

_____

_____

_____

List three ways you constructively let out your anger.

_____

_____

_____

_____

_____

_____

Notes

Chapter VII

Discovering the Secrets of Dreams

"The unending paradox is that we do learn through pain."
- Madeleine L'Engle

"Make your own recovery the first priority in your life."
- Robin Norwood

Studying my dreams during my period of depression proved to be an interesting and beneficial endeavor. For years I had had dreams about houses — long before the terrible Mother's Day, when I learned the truth about Ted's behavior. In my dreams, I was always looking at new houses. I was shopping for or we were in the process of buying or I was moving into a new house. The houses were always much larger and more beautiful than the one in which we lived. These house dreams continued the year Ted and I were in therapy together, and I described them to the therapist.

"A new house means a new life," said the therapist, "Dreaming about a new house means you want your life to change."

"Yes," I thought, "I certainly do."

Looking back even before the therapy, I now see symbolism in a dream I had about a house with beautiful wood paneling and lovely blue tile in an open stairwell. I believe the stairwell symbolized my desire to raise my home to a higher level, to be open and unashamed about my life. Perhaps the blue tile symbolized the peace and serenity which I found lacking in my home. The dreams of bigger houses themselves represented my wish to expand my life, to free it from the limits of my dark suspicions and secrets. At the time of the therapy, however, I was satisfied to realize the dreams suggested how badly I wanted my life to change.

Ted's psychologist also helped me interpret my dream concerning a return to my childhood home. In the dream my parents were dead, as they were in reality, and the house was filled with cobwebs, dust and disarray. My close elderly aunt was my companion in this dream, talking with me about family matters. The therapist explained that the appearance of an older woman in a dream may signify the development of the "sage anima," the older female who represents wisdom in the self. The therapist was pleased for me because the "anima" can lend guidance, and she felt my dream meant I was developing wisdom.

During my joint therapy with Ted I opened my mind to my dreams, making a point to remember and record them. Their richness and variety fascinated me. I made friends with my dreams, and they became more and more vivid. Some nights I had as many as four separate and distinct dreams that I could remember and record. After dreaming I would always awaken refreshed and rested, much more so than after a night's sleep when no dreams seemed to have taken place. After recording my dreams I would think about them and let them lead me.

My new therapist, "Ruth," continued to help me understand my dreams as a healing agent embedded in the most private compartments of my mind. She helped me to interpret several memorable dreams. The most important of these were dreams of reassurance in which I found great strength and healing.

A few months after Ted moved out I had a dream of reassurance from my mother. She came to me in a sort of Mona Lisa pose, with a benevolent smile on her face. In life my mother was not a pretty woman, but in my dream she possessed a stately, composed kind of beauty. She spoke no words, but conveyed a distinct message to me: "You have all the strength and power you need to do whatever you want to do, Emma." I awoke from this dream with a sense of serenity, certain that I would be okay, that things in my life would work out.

Some months later I had an even more reassuring dream. In this dream I sensed a presence that used the right hand to caress my entire body. No gender or sexuality was attached to the presence. Again, no words were spoken, yet once again, a definite message was conveyed: "You will be okay." This message gave me the most powerful feeling of warmth, peace and reassurance I had ever experienced. I awakened and sat up, absolutely positive that there was a presence in my bedroom. However, as I looked around the room, no one was there. I was left with the same feeling of safety I had in the dream about my mother. I knew that I did not have to be so concerned and worried. Things would be okay.

I have often asked myself if this were more than a dream; was it in fact, a spiritual experience? I still don't know. All I know is that the reassurance was so complete that I never doubted it for a moment. I was glad I had opened myself to my dreams, to receive the help that was offered.

Other dreams came as warnings of danger. About a month before my divorce was final I began thinking that perhaps Ted could change after all. Perhaps the divorce was a terrible mistake; maybe we could still make a marriage together if only we would halt the legal proceedings. Then I had a vivid dream: Ted and I were on a hillside in my dream, near our mountain retreat. We saw two holes about four inches in diameter near where we were sitting. Ted threw two rocks at each of the two holes. A rock went into one of the holes, and we saw that it was a den of nonpoisonous snakes. From that den, two snakes came to the entrance, and Ted killed both of them with a claw hammer he held in his hand. I begged him not to kill them, citing their beneficial nature in controlling the mouse population and noticing their lovely pastel coloring. To me they looked soft and beautiful, and I felt it was a shame to kill them. The other hole contained a den of poisonous snakes. They did not appear in my dream, but I felt they were deadly rattlesnakes by an angry aura I sensed emanating from the den.

I awakened from this dream feeling sadness and resignation that Ted had killed the beautiful snakes. Also, I experienced an incidental side effect: after that dream I was never again as afraid of snakes, overcoming a life-long fear. More to the emotional point, the dream also helped me lose my fear of being alone in what I perceived to be a threatening male world.

The most significant aspect of that dream was its symbolism regarding Ted and his life. The dream was full of twos. There were two people, two dens, two rocks thrown, two beautiful snakes and two prongs at the end of the claw hammer. For me, all the twosomes symbolized Ted's Jekyll and Hyde personality: the side of him that was respected and admired that he wanted the world to know, and the dark secret side, which he kept hidden. In the dream, I felt he killed that which was beautiful and positive, just as he had killed the beautiful and positive aspects of our life together. The dream told me that hope was gone, Ted would never change and our chance for a life together was dead. Moreover, Ted was still living a lie, speaking with the forked tongue of a snake.

Another vivid dream of warning contained some of the same symbolism, and occurred a few months later, just after Ted signed some money over to me. The day before this dream I received a very seductive letter from Ted, containing statements concerning the money, and how he did not begrudge signing it over to me. In my dream, Ted and I walked toward our cabin with an older couple, who had been happily married in a compatible, stable relationship for many years. We walked up a steep, rocky, narrow path with a wall of rock on one side. On the other side was a gentle, rocky slope, which led down to a rushing stream. Ted fished as we walked along, repeatedly losing his pole. Each time I found another bough and made him a new pole. The third and last pole I found was forked, but he lost it too. As we walked, we carried various items toward the cabin. Suddenly a purple comforter fell into the stream. Our older male friend attempted to retrieve it, but failed.

"This is very different from ours," the older woman exclaimed as we reached the cabin.

I sobbed and pleaded with Ted. "How can you throw away so much?"

Below us, men in machines shaped like sardine cans were chipping away at the sheer rock wall. As they crashed into the wall their machines nearly tipped over, but they were always able to right themselves. Crashing into the wall, they caused chips to fly from the rock.

When I awoke, I felt nothing. No emotion whatsoever. Later, in therapy, I sobbed uncontrollably. I then saw the contrast between our marriage and the solid marriage of our older friends. I saw how hard I had worked, only to have Ted throw away all we had achieved together. I saw the strange, violent forces that had chipped away at our relationship. There was the forked stick, which once again symbolized Ted's split personality. The lost poles symbolized his lack of focus and need for my assistance. I saw the comfort (the purple comforter) of my marriage thrown and lost into the rushing water. I felt that this dream too, was warning me that Ted would never change and I should abandon any hope for reconciliation.

A few months later, in one other dream of warning, I had planned a Christmas dinner. My table looked beautiful, perfect and complete with bright red ribbons around the water glasses. Ted was late coming home for this special dinner, and when he arrived he was shabbily dressed in an old fur coat and seemed shrunken. In the dream I knew he had gone back to having affairs with other women once again, and I knew that hope was out of the question. In all these dreams of warning, my subconscious told me I should never consider the possibility of resuming life with Ted.

In addition to dreams of reassurance and warning, there is another important category of dreams that influenced me. I call them *dreams of guidance.* During the period of my therapy I had many dreams about doctors, dentists and health professionals who, I believe, were guiding me toward healing. One of the most prominent of these dreams involved a long-time friend who was a pediatrician. In the dream my friend had been called to do a mobile health practice in Upstate New York. He was traveling from town to town to help people take care of their health problems. Knowing I was familiar with the area, he consulted me about various towns and the roads between them so we reviewed maps together. Suddenly, I was in the car with him and traveling about in my home state, but the terrain and plant life were very different from what I had known. I felt quite certain I was in my home state, but I saw that it had changed immensely. At one intersection I looked to the left and saw a lioness. She looked so soft and friendly and gentle I was sure I could have petted her.

"Why, I have seen two other lionesses this week," I remarked to my friend.

For me this dream scenario was highly symbolic of my search for direction. I had my maps and was seeking my way, returning to the location of my roots to find it. I was in the company of a healer, perhaps symbolizing my therapist, who helped me travel a road I knew but which was strangely unfamiliar. The healer wore the guise of a pediatrician because I had reverted to child-like needs in my search. The gentle lioness represented my violent emotions, which had recently become tame and under control. In my mind there were three lionesses and three is considered the number to completion in dream therapy. This suggested that the taming process was finished. I confronted my violent emotions and no longer was afraid of them.

In yet another guidance dream I had moved back to my hometown, ready to open a unique auto service store. I found myself outside my store, marking footprints leading to it when I heard others gossip. "What an attractive person," they whispered, "What a good catch for any man."

I told Ruth about this dream and she was delighted. "Your self-esteem is high," she said. "Traveling in a car is a symbol of high self-esteem. Your self regard is so high that you are planning to take care of other people's self-esteem." She was also pleased about what other people were saying about me in my dream. Because I thought I was a desirable person, I believed other people thought so too.

Studying my dreams helped me to listen to my innermost thoughts, to gain confidence, and to understand that I was progressing in my search for a new life.

Chapter VII Exercise

Carl Jung, world famous Swiss psychologist, believed that dreams contained universal symbols that bore significant messages for us. He knew that understanding and respecting dreams gives us an important opportunity to understand our own unconscious. You write the screenplays for your dreams. These scenarios are a tool for understanding yourself and your life. Use them as an inner resource to recognize assurance, danger and guidance in your life.

1. Write down a dream you remember, with as many details as you can recall: people, colors, places, feelings, words.

_____
_____
_____
_____
_____
_____
_____

2. Write down what you associate with this dream. What comes to your mind?

_____
_____
_____
_____

3. What is your relationship to the words and symbols?

_____
_____
_____
_____
_____
_____

4. Draw a colored picture of one scene from the dream.

5. What do you experience when you look at the picture?

_____
_____
_____
_____
_____

Notes

Chapter VIII

My Secrets to Beginning the Healing Journey as a Single Person

"When I look at the future, it is so bright it burns my eyes."
- Oprah Winfrey

"For over the margins of life comes a whisper, a faint call, a premonition of richer living which we know we are passing by.
Quaker author, Thomas R. Kelly,
A Testament of Devotion

Freedom, freedom, freedom! The word rang in my head and sent a shiver down my spine. I was catapulted back into "singlehood" again. My new state was fraught with fear, but I also felt excited to explore new horizons. I soon learned that freedom comes with many options. How would I step beyond the parameters of the old, familiar box of behaviors and activity that had provided me with identity and security for so long?

I had a panicky feeling that I needed to find a full-time job immediately. The first job I found was with a computer cartridge recycling business. It was a job, but not a good match, as I had little interest in the computer world. While I applauded the company's focus on keeping empty printer cartridges out of the landfill, I could not motivate myself to join the competitive spirit in the office. After a year and a half, when my stress and unhappiness in the position had led to health issues, I knew it was time to leave.

Surprisingly, leaving this first job after my divorce did not feel like failure; rather it felt to me like a survival move, and a sign of moving on and progressing. By spending eighteen months in an inappropriate situation, I learned that my work had to have more meaning. For me, meaning meant working with people in a helping profession.

I had always been attracted to the counseling profession, even psychotherapy. Moving in the direction of those professions meant returning to school for a graduate degree, a prospect that did not appeal to me. An interesting thing happened, however, when I allowed myself to think about going back to school. Everything seemed to fall into place.

In researching possible schools and degree programs, I discovered the College for Social Work at an eastern university. Once I learned more about the program, I decided that this was the place I should consider. I applied to this college program, in fact, the only one which I considered. I shared the news with a friend who also was looking for a career change, and she too, applied. When we were both accepted, we were pleased to be able to make the journey together.

I had made a momentous decision, but many more would spring from that one. First, the College for Social Work was some distance from my established home of 25 years. To make relocation even more complicated the program involved making five more moves during the 27-month program. For the program, three summers would be spent on the campus and two full-time, nine-month internships could be anywhere in the United States. My friend and I requested internships that were in close proximity so we could share living expenses. We felt fortunate when the school honored our requests.

My decision to study such a distance away for eighteen months, left a vacant house back home for me to deal with. I arranged for one daughter to live there while I was gone, with the understanding that I would return home if I were awarded my second internship in my hometown. That arrangement worked out well for the first two years, and my last summer at the university I was able to find a young man to house-sit my home. One big hurdle was satisfactorily overcome.

The next hurdle was financial. I was fortunate to have some financial resources and an independent income. My independent income would not cover all my expenses though, and I wanted to protect my investments and avoid the penalty I would have to pay to withdraw funds. I began by researching lists of scholarships and grants under the category of the "nontraditional" student, but found I did not qualify for any of them.

Then I discovered a sisterhood that focuses on promoting education for women at all socio-economic levels, and made contact. The chapter was eager to sponsor me, and I received a small loan with a very low interest rate. This arrangement was fine for me, as I did not need full financial support. In the course of my research I also discovered that my church had a fund for people going into the ministry or other helping professions, and found that the Department of Social Services could be helpful, especially to people who needed more assistance.

Upon making all the necessary arrangements, I felt euphoric about the change in my situation. I felt strong and eager to meet my new challenge. My friend and I set off in my car, which was loaded to the roof with our necessary clothing and computers for the first summer of graduate school. Our conversations on the long ride were filled with excitement and expectations of our grand adventure.

My first ten-week summer session turned out to offer only slightly less stress than the divorce. I had been a student a very long time ago, and was suddenly confronted with the question of how much strength I had for this adventure. I learned that embarking on my proposed new career involved learning a new vocabulary, reading hour after hour, attending two-hour long class sessions and writing as many as five papers per week. To make matters even more stressful, I had to trot to the end of a long hall to share a bathroom with all the other residents of a dormitory that predated all of us. When my daughter and son-in-law came to attend my graduation, they visited the dorm to see where I had been staying. My son-in-law was incredulous: "You lived *here* for three summers?"

Every activity of my day reminded me that I had made a remarkable change in my life. I was caught up in it, running with it and sometimes feeling as if I were in a fog. However, because of my maturity, I did recognize the value of my life experience, which younger students lacked. Yet it also proved to be both hindrance and help.

When I began my first internship I was able to leave the dorm and settle with my friend and colleague, into a rented condominium. Our new lodgings provided much more normalcy to our lives. There still were papers and projects to be completed for the program, but we had more time for fun and weekend activities. We enjoyed exploring the history-rich New England communities, and I finally felt truly happy. This move was the right thing to do.

I was awarded my final internship in my hometown, performing outpatient psychotherapy in a psychiatric hospital. After one more summer of classes and finishing my thesis, I completed my Masters of Social Work degree. I was 54.

My first position in my new profession was a misfit, and I left after three months. Then the hospital where I had completed my second internship asked me to cover for social workers while they went on vacation. Since I was searching for less than full-time work, that relationship worked out well and has continued for eight years. Now I often work full-time for months, and although the work is not without stress, I find it very rewarding.

I am proud that I was able to go through the rigors of preparing myself for this new profession and to make the transition into it. I am proud of my courage in finally facing what I needed to do in order to lead a whole and healthy life. I am grateful for all the help I received along the way, and that I was wise enough to accept it and to reject what was not helpful. I am eager to share what I have learned on this awesome and painful healing journey. For that sharing I have reserved the last chapter of this book.

Chapter VIII Exercise

Write about the biggest challenge you face right now. What is the most difficult decision that you have to make or need to make? How has your past prepared you for the challenge and the decision?

_____
_____
_____
_____
_____
_____
_____
_____
_____
_____
_____
_____
_____
_____
_____
_____
_____
_____
_____
_____
_____
_____
_____
_____

Notes

Chapter IX

Lessons Learned from My Secrets

"Life shrinks or expands in proportion to one's courage."
- Anais Nin

"You must train your intuition-you must trust the small voice inside you that tells you exactly what to say, what to decide."
- Ingrid Bergman

My story is no longer a secret. I have taken the extraordinary step of revealing my secrets in the hope that readers who identify with some of my experiences may then see in their own lives, symptoms of problems that can be addressed.

My secret was that I was married to a full-blown sex addict whose condition dictated that he resort to ever more risky behavior in order to achieve a satisfactory "high." Another person's relationship experience may involve the sex addict's use of voyeurism, obscene phone calls, pornographic materials in magazines or on a web site, excessive masturbation, child molestation, or any number of other addictive behaviors. A complete list of such behaviors and their levels may be found in Patrick Carnes' book, *Out of the Shadows*. My sincere hope is that my revelations will raise the level of consciousness for others who are in abusive relationships, helping them summon strength and courage to seek a better life.

In my journey from married to single life, from denial to healing, I came to a point of reflection: "What have I learned?" I asked myself.

"Could I have learned these things without going through so much pain?" I wondered.

There is a time for everything

I discovered that there is a time for everything— especially, a time to end a toxic relationship. I found I had given enough time and energy to a situation that was not going to improve. I was exhausted, and had bankrupted my emotional reserves trying for improvement. I do believe that, had I remained any longer in my relationship I might have succumbed to severe mental illness. I do not advocate that anyone remain in a relationship to that point. In addition, I do not look upon my getting out of my relationship as a failure, but rather as a flight to survival. I was at a place where I had to choose for or against my own life. It was time to give myself permission to take another path, to explore where it could take me.

Although I believe that it was time for me to take flight, I probably could not have done so sooner because I was not ready. The expression *"getting your ducks in a row"* describes what I had been doing for some time on an unconscious level. I sensed that before I could trust my wings to carry me I needed a safety net of support. By the time I fled I had already accomplished several things which allowed me to feel more ready to launch into a new life: I had accumulated a group of friends for emotional support; I had inquired about health insurance from my employer; I had satisfied myself that I would have a measure of financial independence.

Be alert to effects on children

Many believe that it is important to keep a family together for the sake of the children. I, too, believed that for a long time. Now I know that staying in my marriage was not a good choice for my daughters; they paid the high price of experiencing our family turmoil.

Most threatening to our four daughters' well-being was that there was an unhealthy role model of husband and father in our house. A sexual tension permeated every action among family members. There was a seductive quality in the father-daughter dynamic, such as in the way they were encouraged by their father to dress inappropriately. The unavoidable message was: "You will be admired and get attention by being seductive." Their father's overt and covert behavior led to decisions by the children to emulate promiscuous sexual behavior and to choose men who played out the same role as their father had.

Our family turmoil resulted in my depression, making it difficult for me to be available to my daughters. Moreover, it made me appear to be disconnected, which they interpreted as my being aloof and uninterested in their lives. Because I had no energy for them, it was easy for them to direct their anger at me.

Twelve years after my divorce another daughter requested that she and I undergo mother-daughter therapy, which proved to be very beneficial. I was overjoyed at her request, as I had been secretly thinking of the same thing, not daring to suggest it. She needed to know that she was loved, but had I suggested therapy earlier, she probably would have rejected the idea. It was important for her to define the place and the time and to recognize the value of therapy. Our treatment lasted for nine months, with the agreement to return for more sessions if either of us felt the need to do so. Our relationship continues to improve, with once-a-month dates for an activity together.

I learned too late that my own mother was suspicious of my husband's behavior around his daughters. Nor was she the only one to observe unusual behavior: friends later reported feeling uncomfortable about what they perceived as inappropriate behavior between the girls and their father. Friends and family who are aware of such behavior must summon the courage to confront the possibilities. It could be extremely important—possibly even lifesaving—for both children and parents.

Experience the emotion

I sensed that I had to feel my distress in order to heal. I knew that I had to let myself experience all the wrenching emotions — pain, sorrow, fear, anguish and anger. Allowing myself to feel all those searing emotions in their full force was cleansing. At the time I was not aware of their value, nor was I conscious of a decision on my part to let my emotions run their course. That awareness came later with therapy.

Immediately after I chose my lawyer and had Ted served with divorce papers, the negative emotions receded for a time. What replaced them was an almost delirious emotional "high." I had made a decision and taken action. The nightmare that was my life was about to be transformed. I still couldn't sleep, but now it was because I felt too euphoric.

Negative emotions quickly returned when I faced the reality of hours of attorneys' conferences and haggling about the property settlement. Also, I was faced with dealing directly with Ted. My nightmare still had quite a long way to go, but the process was underway.

During this period I began to learn how to deal with emotional pain. I learned that running away from the suffering is pointless. The only meaningful response was to embrace the pain, appreciate it and understand it. The journey of healing begins when one engages in solidarity with pain. Curative powers become available when one connects with the pain inside one's innermost being.

Be aware of mind, body and spirit as parts of the whole person

I believe that the mind, body and spirit are a whole, and when one part of that whole is under stress the other parts are compromised. For example, I recognized a physical problem to be a cue that my job at the time was not right for me and was damaging my health.

An even more serious illness eventually arose. Imagine my shock when the nurse motioned me back to the x-ray room to repeat a mammogram. A suspicious spot was discovered. Within a week I had an ultrasound and a needle biopsy, and was diagnosed with breast cancer. Though I cannot prove my breast cancer was a result of stress, I remain convinced that the extreme stress I experienced was a contributor in compromising my immune system.

Dependence to independence is a slow evolution

I discovered that my move to a satisfying, independent life evolved slowly, and that it actually had been in process for many years prior to my divorce. As with so many women of my generation, I went from my father's house to my husband's house without ever tasting the freedom of being on my own. I had missed out on the exhilarating (and frightening) experience of taking care of myself, of facing the world and making my own decisions.

The year I discovered my husband's first affair was also the year my father had a severe stroke and was not expected to live. At age 39, I was faced with the reality that the two men in my life I had depended on the most could leave me in the same year. The reality hit me like a bolt of lightning, and I paid attention. I began to focus on enhancing my independence, and worked on it for the next ten years.

My first step toward independence occurred when I was offered a position as director of the Christian Education Department at my church. I took the job, though Ted opposed it. In this position I gained a great deal of self-confidence as colleagues recognized and encouraged my talents. My creative, organizational, leadership and teaching skills were unleashed and they flourished. In addition, my spiritual life was enriched through attending and leading workshops in religious education.

I had always been very focused on my "female/anima," nurturing qualities, and my new position allowed me to continue those kinds of activities. It also offered me a measure of financial and professional independence, to bring out the "male/animus" side of my personality. The bringing together of the female and male sides of the personality allows a person to perform any tasks that society labels either masculine or feminine.

As my animus developed, I began to demonstrate an enterprising spirit, courage, truthfulness and confidence in my spirituality. I became more assertive about taking care of myself, allowing myself things that I wanted but had sacrificed for what I thought was the good of the family.

These early steps were valuable in helping me later to understand and accept my own worth, as well as to enhance my ability to succeed with my developing independence.

Redefine yourself, but enjoy the moment

When my world changed to that of a divorced woman, I knew I had to redefine myself from my old life as a wife, mother and part-time employee. My first reaction was to try to prove myself by pushing very hard. I went out into the world determined to do something that would make the rest of my life more meaningful. I enrolled for graduate school. It had always been my desire to earn a graduate degree, but before the divorce it had seemed more important for my spouse to attain that next degree and for me to support his needs and the needs of our children.

After I earned my graduate degree, it was very important for me to find work that held some prestige. For me, *"prestige"* involved work that held great meaning, work that involved relationships and contributing to society. I was aware that I possessed helping, healing and teaching capabilities to share with others.

It was about ten years after the dissolution of my marriage that I was finally able to give myself permission to relax and not to struggle so hard. I found I could work less and even search for a less stressful position. I no longer needed to drive myself, to prove myself successful. I had, in fact, at last truly redefined myself, and it was a satisfying definition.

Marriage can reflect other relationships

"Why had I married a man who was never emotionally available?" I asked myself. Had I married this man in order to work out my relationship with my mother, my father, or both? Was I repeating a childhood pattern?

I examined my relationship with my father. He was the other most significant man in my life, and I realized I had no idea who he was. I cannot remember ever having a meaningful, intimate conversation with him. We never shared any feelings, thoughts or ideas with each other.

What of my image of my mother? I remember her as an angry woman who worked all the time. When I was about twelve years of age, my younger brother was killed in a farm accident. My mother became severely depressed by the loss of a child. From then on I grew up as an only child with two unavailable parents.

Did I choose my marriage relationship because it felt familiar and comfortable, conforming with the role model I had for relationships? Harville Hendrix, author of *Keeping the Love You Find and Getting the Love You Want,* believes we continue in relationships to work out wounds from our childhood. Lending credence to Mr. Hendrix' theory, I chose a man who turned out to be unavailable for intimacy and closeness just like my parents.

Conversely, perhaps I was searching for the intimacy and closeness I did not get from my parents, believing Ted could provide that. As a young person, I was shy and quiet, finding it difficult to enter new situations easily. Ted was gregarious and at ease in crowds of strangers when I first met him. During the course of our marriage, and as my confidence grew as an adult, I found I no longer had to stand behind my husband — or a door—in unfamiliar circumstances. By the end of our relationship, our roles had reversed, and I became the outgoing, socially accomplished partner.

Ultimately I recognized that this man had seduced something within me. A sexual seduction in his eyes was at the same time attractive and repulsive to me. Eventually, I learned that the one I believed could complement my personality and meet my needs was, in fact, perpetuating my deepest needs and fears.

Listen to your intuition

I have learned that I possess good intuitive sense, along with strong logical and intellectual capabilities. There were many times when I would attempt to listen to my intuition and begin to question my husband's behavior. At these times he would convince me that I was wrong or that I was not thinking clearly.

"You do not know what the real world is like. Everyone behaves this way," he told me. Perhaps because of my lack of early experience and somewhat protected childhood, I did not feel I could refute this. But intuitively I knew he was wrong.

For a long time I subjugated my intuitive sense, pushing it aside because I did not have faith in it. Had I paid attention to intuition earlier in my life, I might not have married the person I did. Later I "knew" there was something wrong, or at least not quite right, about my relationship with Ted, but I chose to ignore my intuition. I believed that by working harder and harder on it I could make the relationship work. With my intuitive sense shoved deep down so it wouldn't function, I could not identify what was wrong with my marriage relationship or with Ted's personality. I should have enlisted the help of the intuitive side of my being.

Seek community

All my life I have always sought out community. My primary community has generally been the church, but several groups have provided comfort, perspective, support, confidence, and opportunity for growth. "Where two or three are gathered in my name, there I am also," was the Biblical text that carried me through many difficult days.

My community of friends turned out to be essential during my struggle through pain to successful independence. On my bad days I would plead with friends, "Please don't give up on me. I will get better." Those who themselves had been in hard places knew I would eventually feel better. Others just loved me, stuck with me in the bad times, and stayed with me through to the good.

Notes

Epilogue

Over twelve years ago this book began as a work of emotional catharsis for me. It has been difficult to write, even wrenching at times. The finished product did not evolve in a linear fashion, but with many revisions and times of reworking and rethinking. For long periods, sometimes years, it lay in a box in a dark closet. Even then, although it was out of my sight, it remained my dream.

This book and its subject never left me; partly because I knew there were others dealing with the same issues, partly because I knew there were few books to help me in my time of need. Over the years, friends would ask how my *"project"* was progressing. One in particular would say, "It needs to be in print to help others."

As you finish reading this book, I hope you have gained new insights and perspectives into sexual addiction and its effect, if so, then I will have accomplished my goal.

My purpose in writing and publishing this book is to raise awareness, in both the sex addicts and those in their world. More than simply raising awareness, I hope to provide special focus on the plight of the partner of the sexual addict, to offer information as well as hope to those who find themselves in such relationships.

If you or your partner are exhibiting some of the symptoms discussed in this book, I hope you will consider whether you are in an abusive relationship. If you are in such a relationship, I hope you will work toward changes within it or get out of it. You, too, can discover that there is a better, more fulfilling way to live. The path to a different life may have ruts that tend to steer you back into the same old track. The joy and freedom of a different kind of life are worth every effort to find new directions. I cannot imagine returning to the way I was living. I feel younger, freer, livelier, busier, healthier and happier.

You can too.

Look for the Symptoms

If you find yourself exhibiting a number of the following symptoms, you may be collaborating in an emotionally abusive relationship with a sex addict, or any kind of addict.

- Denying anything is wrong
- High stress in the home
- Concealing behavior of the addict
- Alibis, excuses and justification to others
- Overlooking addict's behavior
- Rationalizing addict's behavior
- On-going list of resentments and disappointments in the relationship
- Feelings of depression and remorse
- Deterioration of family life
- Growing self-doubt and fear
- Unusual dreams
- Increasing financial problems
- Over-extension and over-involvement in work or outside activities
- Believing you can change addict's behavior
- Protecting the addict from consequences of behavior
- Failed efforts to confront the addict with his or her "problem"
- Fantasizing and obsessing about the addict's problem
- Feeling unique or alone with the problem
- Thought of suicide or suicide attempts
- Doubting your intuitive feelings

For more information, visit the web site for Sex Addicts Anonymous, www.sexaa.org or contact S-Anon, a support group for families, at 615-833-3152.

Bibliography

Carnes, Patrick. **OUT OF THE SHADOWS; UNDERSTANDING SEXUAL ADDICTION,** Minneapolis: CompCare Publications, 1983.

Carnes, Patrick. **CONTRARY TO LOVE,** Minneapolis, CompCare Publications, 1989.

Dawson, Emma.**SPOUSES/PARTNERS OF SEX ADDICTS: PHYSICAL, EMOTIONAL & SEXUAL ABUSE IN FAMILIES OF ORIGIN.** Master's Thesis, 1992.

Fischer, Kathleen.**WOMEN AT THE WELL, FEMINIST PERSPECTIVES ON SPIRITUAL DIRECTION.** New York, Paulist Press, 1988.

Hendrix, Harville. **GETTING THE LOVE YOU WANT: A GUIDE FOR COUPLES.** New York, Harper & Row Publishers, 1988.

Jung, Carl G. **MAN AND HIS SYMBOLS.** New York, Doubleday & Company Inc., 1964.

Sanford, John **A. THE INVISIBLE PARTNERS.** New York, Paulist Press, 1980.

Carnes, Patrick, Griffin, Elizabeth, Delmonico, David, Moriarty, Joseph. **IN THE SHADOWS OF THE NET: BREAKING FREE OF COMPULSIVE ONLINE SEXUAL BEHAVIOR.** Minnesota Hazelden Information Education, 2001.

Schneider, Jennifer, Weiss, Robert. **CYBERSEX EXPOSED: SIMPLE OR OBSESSION?.** Minnesota, Hazelden Publishing and information, 2001.

Notes

Printed in France by Amazon
Brétigny-sur-Orge, FR

30656857R00080